The Fast Track Detox Diet

The Fast Track Detox Diet

Ann Louise Gittleman, PhD

C
—

Century · London

Published by Century in 2005

1 3 5 7 9 10 8 6 4 2

Copyright © Ann Louise Gittleman 2005

Ann Louise Gittleman has asserted her right under the Copyright,
Designs and Patents Act, 1988 to be identified as the author of this work

Published simultaneously in the US in 2005 by Broadway,
a division of the Random House Group Inc.

First published in the United Kingdom in 2005 by Century
The Random House Group Limited
20 Vauxhall Bridge Road, London SW1V 2SA

Random House Australia (Pty) Limited
20 Alfred Street, Milsons Point, Sydney,
New South Wales 2061, Australia

Random House New Zealand Limited
18 Poland Road, Glenfield
Auckland 10, New Zealand

Random House South Africa (Pty) Limited
Endulini, 5a Jubilee Road, Parktown 2193, South Africa

The Random House Group Limited Reg. No. 954009
www.randomhouse.co.uk

A CIP catalogue record for this book is available from the British Library

Papers used by Random House are natural, recyclable products
made from wood grown in sustainable forests. The manufacturing processes
conform to the environmental regulations of the country of origin

Typeset by SX Composing DTP, Rayleigh, Essex
Printed and bound in Germany by
GGP Media GmbH, Pößneck

Contents

Get on the Fast Track!

*Each progressive spirit is opposed by a thousand
mediocre minds appointed to guard the past.*

– MAURICE MAETERLINCK

What if you could lose 1.35 to 3.6 kg/3 to 8 lb in a single day?

What if that nearly instant weight loss made you feel lighter, freer, cleaner and more energised?

What if that one day of weight loss could help jump-start a long-term weight-loss plan? What if that single day began a healing, cleansing, revitalising process, raising your awareness of the poisons that pollute our environment and purging your body of the toxins that set you up for weight gain, fatigue, and a host of deadly, debilitating diseases?

Well, that single day is here. It's called the Fast Track Detox Diet. It's safe. It feels terrific. And it works.

A One-Day Miracle Diet:
Too Good to Be True?

Who doesn't like quick fixes and magic bullets? They're the reason that weight-loss products promising instant results have become a multibillion-dollar industry that's growing every year. The fact that most of these trendy diets don't work, don't last and often put us at risk of serious health problems seems less important to many desperate dieters than the glittering promises these plans make.

As a nutritional maverick, I have always bucked the system. Yet for more than twenty years, even I believed that there was no such thing as a magic bullet – although my internationally bestselling *Fat Flush Plan* had certainly come close! Throughout my hands-on experience with thousands of patients and clients in the public health arena (including a stint as the chief nutritionist for the paediatric clinic at New York City's Bellevue Hospital) and in the private sector (several years as the director of nutrition at the Pritikin Longevity Center in Santa Monica, California), I've always advocated long-term lifestyle changes, avoiding the one-shot answers that seem so popular in the weight-loss world. Although many diet gurus preached the gospel of exercising more and eating less, of cutting out fats, or – more recently – of eliminating carbs, I've always understood that our bodies and metabolisms are too complex for such simple solutions.

When I introduced my two-week programme in *Beyond Pritikin* nearly two decades ago and then brought out a more extensive version of that diet in *The Fat Flush Plan*, I helped revolutionise weight loss by introducing the concept of detox to the diet world. Years before Atkins, South Beach and the Zone, I predicted that the low-fat, high-carb diets so popular in the 1980s were actually creating weight gain, sugar cravings, fatigue and diabetes – health concerns that have taken on epidemic proportions today. I was the first to point out the importance of the essential fatty acids for weight loss as well as for overall health and beauty, a recurring theme in my two dozen books. My millions of readers around the world, and the millions more who visit my website (www.fasttrackdetox.com) have always known that they can count on me for sound, well-researched nutritional advice based on both real-life experience and scientific evidence.

Then, in November 2003, *Woman's World* magazine came to me with an unusual request. They wanted a one-day juice fast, the recipe for a special brew that would enable readers to quickly lose 1.35 to 2.25 kg/3 to 5 lb so they could fit into that special outfit or take off that holiday weight.

A fast can be a terrific weight-loss method because, during a fast, the primary source of fuel for the cells is fat. Of course, I'd known for years that an improperly done fast can actually sabotage weight loss by disrupting your metabolism. The wrong kind of fasting can also threaten your health by stressing your liver, clogging your colon and flooding your bloodstream with the oil-soluble toxins that your body had been storing in its fat.

On the other hand, a fast done correctly – with your body prepared for fasting and properly supported during the regime – can flush the accumulated toxins from your cells, accelerate your weight loss, cleanse your body and combat the effects of ageing. Periodic fasting of this type can clear up skin conditions, boost your energy and put a sparkle in your eyes.

Moreover, a properly done fast offers you a chance to detoxify your body. A body overloaded with toxins and pollutants suffers from a weakened immune system, a stressed-out liver and, in all probability, a malfunctioning colon. Such 'toxic' bodies are far more vulnerable to disorders great and small, ranging from colds, flu and fatigue to arthritis, asthma and allergies – all the way up to autoimmune conditions, heart disease and cancer. In other words, *properly done fasting is the missing link to better health.*

And fasting and detox have one more benefit, perhaps the most dramatic and least well known of all. *Fasting is the missing link to long-term weight loss.* That's because detox and weight loss go hand in hand. So the more toxic your body becomes, the more difficulty you will have losing weight and keeping it off.

Weight Loss and Toxicity: The Missing Link

The connection between weight loss and toxicity is so important, I'll say it again: *The more toxic your body becomes, the more difficulty you'll have losing weight.* Does that sound like an extreme statement? Then consider for a moment the 'obesity epidemic' that you've no doubt read about. We now know that more than sixty diseases have been linked to obesity. Three-quarters of British adults are overweight, while 22 per cent of us are officially obese. The number of obese children has tripled in the last twenty years, with 10 per cent being classed thus, rising to 17 per cent of fifteen-year-olds. Think of it – a whopping seven out of ten Britons face a weight gain that might literally kill them by setting them up for diabetes, heart disease and other fatal conditions.

Now recall the almost daily warnings about the growing amount of pollutants, toxins and synthetic chemicals in our food, water and air. The average person in Britain each year consumes 5 kg/11 lb of food additives and has 4.5 litres/1 gallon of pesticides and herbicides sprayed on the fruit and vegetables they eat. Our cows, sheep, chickens and pigs are injected with oestrogens to fatten them up and then stuffed with pesticide-laden grains to satisfy their artificial hunger.

Well, I'm here to tell you that there's a connection. Based on my twenty years as a practising nutritionist, I see a clear link between rising levels of obesity and the fact that most of us are becoming more toxic every year.

1. **Our bodies are staggering under the enormous load of industrial toxins that have entered our food, water and environment – and these toxins are making us fat.** First, we ingest the hormone-laden foods meant to fatten cattle, sheep and

chicken up for market. Then our hormones are further disrupted by the pesticides, chemical fertilisers and heavy metals that these poor animals consume with their feed. Finally, our poor polluted planet bombards us with new toxic invaders every day, from the methyl mercury in our fish to the solvents in our acrylic nails. These toxins are in our homes, our workplace, our cosmetics and our food. They're deadly to our health and disastrous for our weight.

2. **Most of us eat far less fibre than we need and consume far more sugar, refined flour, saturated fats and protein than we should.** In this toxic era, we need fibre more than ever, to help us neutralise the toxins and scrub them out of our system. A diet rich in whole grains, legumes, fruit and fresh vegetables offers us plenty of fibre – but how many of us eat that way? We're more likely to consume fatty, sugary and flour foods or to go on the low-carb, low-fibre diets like Atkins and South Beach. Rural Africans eat about 55 grams of dietary fibre a day, compared to the UK average intake of 22 grams. The average Briton also eats less fruit and veggies than almost any other European. So the food we eat sits in our colons for weeks, months, even years, where it slowly putrefies, bloating our stomachs and poisoning our bodies. Our poor, overloaded livers are supposed to detoxify our bodies, but they can't keep up with this toxic challenge. They do

the best they can, but how can they properly metabolise fat when they're assaulted by this daily dose of toxins? Once again, we gain weight.

3. **Low-carb diets are adding new stresses to our liver, colon and entire digestive system.** Some people can lose weight on low-carb diets – I'll be the first to admit it. But the long-term consequences of low-carb diets can be disastrous for both health and long-term weight loss. First, low-carb diets like Atkins and South Beach steer dieters towards high-protein foods such as beef, chicken, fish and pork – the very foods simply loaded with the toxins we've just discussed. Then they urge dieters to avoid the fibre-rich fruit and vegetables that might help purify and eliminate those toxins. Finally, they load us up with so many proteins that we can't produce enough stomach acid to digest them all. Stress, vitamin and mineral deficiencies, and poor eating habits have already deprived most of us of the stomach acid we need. So we end up with an acid reflux epidemic while the undigested meat and cheese rots right there in our gut, overloading our liver and intestines with such poisons as indican, ammonia, cadaverine and histidine. And, you guessed it, our weight continues to rise.

Clearly, we are sorely in need of both *diet and detox* – a safe, effective way to lose weight based on supporting our livers and colons. Maybe, I thought, the one-day weight-loss miracle that *Woman's World* had requested would allow me to kill two birds with one stone. With the right fast, dieters could lose significant amounts of weight virtually overnight, and they could also take advantage of fasting's age-old ability to cleanse and purify our bodies. A one-day fast would give both men and women a sense of how satisfying good nutrition and cellular cleansing can be. People who successfully completed a properly done fast might even move on to long-term lifestyle changes.

The key would be to develop a fast that provided dieters with adequate nutritional support, particularly for their livers and colons – our major detox organs. So I drew on my years of research, writing and counselling to come up with a plan. The results were astounding.

The Fast Track Detox Diet: A Proven System

First, the one-day fast I developed did indeed achieve immediate weight-loss results. *Woman's World* readers reported losing 1.4, 1.8, 2.25 kg/3, 4, 5 lb in a single day. The special 'miracle juice' I created for dieters to drink while they fasted successfully staved off hunger pangs, maintained metabolism and provided the nutritional back-up fasters need to support their livers and colons.

But my fast went far beyond simple weight loss. It also allowed dieters to taste the delights of detox, the enormous health benefits we can achieve by ridding our bodies of the toxins that bog them down.

Sure enough, the first people who tried my fast reported quick weight loss, no hunger and vastly increased energy.

So I expanded the *Woman's World* plan, creating an entirely new way to combine weight loss and detox. This book is the result.

Losing Weight, Gaining Energy

As I started to come up with an improved and expanded version of Fast Track, I believed that my new plan would continue to offer the dramatic benefits that *Woman's World* readers had experienced with the earlier programme. But like any good clinician, I wanted to test my hypothesis. So I shared this developing detox programme with my own Fat Flushers as well as with more than a hundred dieters in Syracuse, New York, under the guidance of a registered dietitian. The Syracuse group was composed of men and women aged sixteen to seventy, all of whom had struggled for a long time with weight loss and health eating.

And the programme worked! In fact, the results were even better than my initial estimates, causing me to revise my prediction of the upper limit of one-day weight loss from 2.25 to 3.6 kg/5 to 8 lb.

Most striking was the experience of Michael Pankhurst, a fifty-eight-year-old who had struggled with his weight throughout his life. Before starting the one-day fast, he pronounced himself 'dubious'. But by the end of the day, his doubts had vanished with his fat.

'I lost eight pounds,' he enthused. 'My mental clarity during the day was greatly improved. So was my energy level, despite a pre-existing throat condition. And I wasn't even hungry. I think I will try to do it frequently, to boost mental clarity and weight loss.'

As Michael discovered, the benefits of the *Fast Track Detox Diet* went far beyond weight. Other dieters experienced the same lightness, energy and mental clarity that the *Woman's World* dieters had felt. They also reported that the Fast Track got them back on track for healthy eating, enabled them to shed extra Christmas and holiday weight, and helped them break their dieting plateau. They were impressed with their greater alertness, glowing skin, sparkling eyes and toned, tight feeling. Many of them told me that they wanted to make the Fast Track a special ritual or a regular part of their routine – once a month or during the change of season – to regain that cleansed, energised feeling and sense of emotional and physical well-being. (And some of them, too, reported better sex after cleansing!)

I also noticed that some of the Syracuse fasters experienced some symptoms – headache, irritability, fatigue – that I knew resulted from caffeine addiction and insufficient liver support from their previous diet. With what I learned from their experience, I went on to design the expanded, fully supportive programme that you see in this book.

The Fast Track: A Three-Stage Process

Thanks to my own clinical trials, I can assure you that the Fast Track is both an effective weight-loss plan and a superb detox system, a simple, easy and effective way to lose weight and get your health back on the *fast* track.

What distinguishes the *Fast Track Detox Diet* from all those other plans out there? Well, for one thing, although you will almost certainly lose between 1.4 and 3.6 kg/3 and 8 lb in a single day, you don't just subject your body into a fast unprepared. You spend an entire week on the Seven-Day Prequel, eating the Liver-Loving Foods that your body's major detox organ so desperately needs. You'll also load up on Colon-Caring Foods to help your colon purge the toxins and waste from your body.

Then, after the fast is over, you'll seal in the results with a Three-Day Sequel that includes liver and colon support along with special natural food sources of *probiotics* – fermented foods that support the friendly bacteria your system needs to synthesise vitamins and promote immune function.

FAST TRACK: THE ONE-DAY DETOX DIET

Stage One: Seven-Day Prequel
Nourish yourself with *Liver-Loving* and *Colon-Caring* Foods to fortify your major detox and elimination organs during your one-day fast.

Stage Two: One-Day Fast

Fast for a single day while drinking a delicious, spiced Miracle Juice, specially designed to stave off hunger pangs, boost your metabolism, keep your blood sugar steady and flush toxins from your system.

Stage Three: Three-Day Sequel

Ease back into eating with more *Liver-Loving* and *Colon-Caring* Foods to flush any remaining toxins from your system. Consume foods rich in probiotics, which will support the friendly bacteria that keep your digestion and immune system working at peak efficiency.

CHAPTER
2

Why You Need This Book

*Man is more the product of his environment
than of his genetic endowment.*

– RENÉ JULES DUBOS

I'll never forget it.

I was giving a workshop for the Learning Annex in San Francisco when I made what I thought was an offhand reference to the relationship between weight loss and the environment.

'Of course, living in a toxic world is probably our biggest single obstacle to losing weight,' I told this group of veteran dieters, many of whom were there precisely because they expected me to offer some new suggestions for the weight loss they'd struggled with for so many frustrating years. 'When our bodies are assaulted by so many pesticides, petroleum-based fertilisers, additives, preservatives, antibiotics, hormones and environmental pollutants, that's bad for our health, of course – but it also makes it much harder to lose weight and keep it off.'

I was about to move on to my next point when I was interrupted by a sea of waving hands. 'Wait just a minute,' said one woman in her late twenties, who later told me she'd been a runner, and a dieter, since her teenage years. 'I know pollution is bad for our bodies in general, sure, everybody knows that. But how does it affect our weight?' The emphatically nodding heads across the room told me that she was far from the only dieter puzzled about this connection.

Well, I told her, the liver is your body's filter, charged with neutralising all sorts of substances from the waste products of everyday metabolism to the ever increasing load of toxins from our air, water, food, cosmetics and workplace. One of the most serious results of an over-stressed or toxic liver is that it becomes so bogged down, it can't fully metabolise fat. As a result, it dumps fat and cholesterol back into the bloodstream, sabotaging your weight loss and putting you at risk of numerous health problems, including indigestion, fatigue, high chole-sterol, depression, mood swings, lupus, arthritis and other autoimmune conditions. A toxic liver also creates disastrous results for your skin, leaving you with a tendency to blotchy patches, 'liver spots' and rashes.

Meanwhile, your colon – designed to eliminate both natural bodily waste and toxins – is likewise labouring under a double strain. If you're not getting enough fibre, and most of us aren't, especially if you're on a low-carb diet, your colon doesn't have the support it needs to do its job. An overworked colon means that toxins and bile (a crucial substance produced by the liver) can sit in your gut too long. Eventually, your body reabsorbs the toxins and sends them back to the liver once again.

'And that's just the health side of the picture,' I told my increasingly horrified listeners. 'I can also tell you that wastes left in the colon can harden and create impactions that cause the colon to expand, resulting in added weight to your abdominal area. That's not fat, it's leftover food and waste products.'

In other words, I concluded, a toxic liver and a clogged colon will sabotage a healthy eating plan faster than a double-dip ice-cream cone! What's the point of struggling to manage our food intake if our organs are giving way under the strain of processing a toxic overload?

Now the interruption came from an older woman's insistently waving hand. She looked to be in her mid-forties, a tall, striking woman who seemed tired and discouraged. Although I could see that she'd worked hard at keeping her weight down, I was struck by her blotchy skin and the dark circles around her eyes. Her scales might be giving her the answers she wanted, but her mirror definitely wasn't.

'How do we know if toxins are our problem?' she asked breathlessly, and again, her neighbours nodded. 'Because I'll tell you, I eat lots of fruit and veggies, so I know I'm getting my fibre. I've given up sugar, except maybe once or twice a week. I'm not on any medications, and I drink a few glasses of wine a month, at most.

But I'm still having trouble keeping the weight off. And I'm tired all the time.'

I ended up meeting with this woman privately and helping her identify the toxins lurking in her diet and her environment: the pesticide-laden strawberries she had each morning for breakfast, the mercury-ridden fish she had been so good about eating five times a week, the hidden toxins in her cosmetics, and the mercury in her fillings. Although not everyone is equally sensitive to these toxic triggers, this woman was – and you may be, too. I told her about some relatively simple ways of detoxing her body, her diet and her home, techniques that I'll share with you throughout this book.

But first things first. By now you're probably wondering if you, too, are suffering from toxic overload that is sabotaging your weight loss, masking your natural beauty and threatening your health. Luckily for us, the body never lies. Once you learn how to read the clues your body is giving you, you can take the necessary steps through the Fast Track to find natural and non-prescription solutions for those symptoms that concern you the most.

Read Your Body Like a Book: Signs of Distress

1. Do you have . . .

   . . . acne, blemishes, hives or itchy rashes?

   . . . discoloration in the eyes?

. . . red, swollen or teary eyes?

. . . haemorrhoids or varicose veins?

. . . hormonal imbalances, such as PMS, menstrual problems, or menopausal concerns, particularly hot flushes?

. . . heat in the upper body, such as a warm face or hot eyes?

. . . light-coloured stools?

. . . gas, bloating, belching and nausea, especially after eating fatty foods?

. . . difficulty digesting fats?

. . . mild frontal headaches after fatty meals?

. . . tendency to loss of appetite or eating disorder?

. . . weight gain, particularly when you are controlling your food intake?

. . . feelings of tiredness or sleepiness after eating?

. . . tendency to wake between 1 am and 3 am?

. . . weak tendons, ligaments or muscles?

. . . pain under the right shoulder blade?

. . . excessive, unexplained or sudden bursts of anger, irritability or rage?

. . . depression, particularly depression unrelated or disproportionate to life events?

. . . elevated liver enzymes (SGOT, SGPT)?

. . . high bilibrubin levels?

* **Regardless of whether you have one or ten of these symptoms, your body is trying to give you an SOS. Whether your symptoms are PMS, discoloured stools, waking up between 1 am and 3 am or any of the other symptoms, your capacity to detox may be impaired and you may be suffering from a sluggish or toxic liver. You will definitely need to build up your liver before the *Fast Track Detox Diet* and support your liver after the One-Day Fast, so don't skip the Seven-Day Prequel or the Three-Day Sequel, both of which include a nutritional strategy for a healthy liver.**

2. *Do you have . . .*

. . . bad breath or an offensive body odour?

. . . a frequent bitter taste in your mouth?

. . . a coated tongue?

. . . putrid and/or painful gas?

. . . digestive disorders?

. . . problems with elimination?

. . . constipation or diarrhoea?

. . . long, thin or foul-smelling stools; stools with undigested food particles?

. . . lower back pain?

. . . abdominal discomfort or fullness?

. . . rectal itching?

. . . bruises that don't heal?

. . . difficulty perspiring?

. . . joint aches and pains?

. . . arthritis?

. . . colitis or diverticulitis?

. . . systematic yeast infections or problems with candida?

. . . parasites or worms?

. . . multiple allergic response syndrome (MARS)?

. . . multiple food allergies or sensitivities to the environment (perfumes, other fragrances, car fumes or other odours)?

* Again, your body is sending you a cry for help with even one of these symptoms, which could indicate impaired elimination and a toxic or sluggish colon. Whether your symptoms are a coated tongue, constipation, candida infection or any of the other symptoms, you will definitely need to stimulate your ability to eliminate waste, so don't skip the Seven-Day Prequel or the Three-Day Sequel, both of which include a nutritional strategy for a healthy colon.

Warning: Toxic Signs Ahead

In addition to the symptoms we've just listed, you might notice many other signs of toxic overload that indicate the need for the One-Day Detox Diet:

- Frequent coughs
- Stuffy nose
- Sinus problems
- A tendency to colds and flu
- Exhaustion, lethargy and fatigue
- Mental dullness or poor memory
- Premature ageing

And if you have trouble losing weight or maintaining your ideal weight, even when you regulate your food intake and exercise regularly, you should definitely consider whether a toxic liver or colon is part of the problem.

Now, if you've taken this quiz and are feeling a bit overwhelmed by the results, don't despair. The bad news is the extent to which toxic substances in our food, air, water and environment are damaging our health and sabotaging our weight loss. But the good news is how much we can do about it. By undertaking the Seven-Day Prequel, One-Day Fast and Three-Day Sequel, you can start right away to support your system and help your body eliminate that toxic build-up.

Low-Carb Diets:
Making the Problem Worse

My client Mercedes was concerned. She'd come to me because she'd started experiencing a host of disturbing symptoms: acne, haemorrhoids, rectal itching, gas, bloating and constipation. Her skin tone wasn't good, and she didn't have the energy she was used to. Her fingernails were starting to peel, chip and break more frequently, and she'd noticed that more hair than usual was coming out in the shower. Plus she felt tired, dragged-out and cranky. When I asked Mercedes about her eating habits, she explained that she'd been on a very low-carb, high-protein diet for about six months. That was another source of frustration, she told me: when it came time to start adding some carbohydrates back into her diet, her weight had immediately begun to creep up.

I told Mercedes that many of her symptoms, were, in my view, signs of toxicity – the inevitable result of the twentieth-century environmental assaults you've just read about. Just think, I told her, industry introduces more than a thousand brand-new chemicals into the atmosphere each year, that's something like three new chemicals a day.

To make matters worse, these pesticides and new chemicals are not just your run-of-the-mill pollutants. They are that special breed known as xenoestrogens, which duplicate some of the effects of oestrogen, the female hormone. They work their way into our food, cosmetics, homes and workplaces, where they disrupt our hormones and increase our weight, besides producing the ugly and unpleasant symptoms she had just described.

Mercedes's problem was further compounded by her high-protein, low-carb diet, which had loaded her up with the most toxic food source of all – hormone- and pesticide-laden animal proteins. At the same time, her regime had deprived her of the fruit, vegetables and whole grains whose fibre vitamins, minerals and antioxidants she desperately needed to fight those toxins. To restore both her health and her ability to lose weight, Mercedes would have to detoxify, supporting her liver and colon so that they could expel the poisons from her system.

Mercedes agreed to try the *Fast Track Detox Diet*, fortifying her liver, unclogging her stagnant colon and starting to clear her body of the poisons she had accumulated. When I saw her two weeks later, the difference was apparent. Her skin had started to clear, her hair had already begun to feel thicker, and her nails had grown in strong and hard. She'd lost 1.8 kg/4 lb on the Fast Track, and she was optimistic about continuing to lose weight with this new approach to eating. Best of all, she told me, she'd regained her normal energy levels, and maybe even a little bit more.

'I don't think I realised how much all that protein on my low-carb diet was weighing me down,' she said. 'Even though I was losing weight, I *felt* heavy, somehow. Now, I feel clean.'

Toxic Invaders: How Low-Carb Dieting Puts Us at Risk

It's a well-known fact: the highest concentration of pesticides and other toxins in our diet comes from meat and dairy products. That's because animals store toxins the same place we do – in their fat. When we eat these polluted animals and their by-products, we are consuming the poisons that they were exposed to, in their feed, in their grazing area and in their toxin-laden farm environment.

Now, I would never counsel you to give up meat, cheese or eggs. On the contrary, high-quality sources of these animal proteins are a mainstay of the Fast Track, as you will see later. But low-carb diets go to the other extreme. Their overemphasis on animal proteins, and their complete lack of consciousness about the need to choose organic meats, 'clean' fish and hormone-free dairy, puts you at increased risk from the toxic invaders you read about above.

As we have seen, conventional animals feeds are among the crops sprayed most heavily with pesticides, herbicides and fungicides. These agricultural chemicals have potentially toxic effects as well as tending to disrupt our hormones and interfere with weight loss. Thus up to 95 per cent of all pesticide residues are found in meat and dairy products. So eating lots of meat, eggs and dairy products – especially if you're not choosing organic foods – hugely increases your exposure to toxins.

Moreover, low-carb diets are sadly lacking in

phytonutrients, crucial food elements found only in fresh fruit and vegetables. Plant foods are rich in antioxidants – vitamins, minerals and other nutritional elements that fight *oxidative stress*, in which cells are destroyed, the immune system is weakened, inflammation occurs and ageing accelerates. As we'll see in Chapter 3, your liver needs big-time antioxidant support to sustain the body's major detoxification pathways. If you're focusing on pesticide- and hormone-laden meats while avoiding cleansing fruit and veggies, you're setting yourself up for a toxic invasion.

Low-carb plans that steer dieters away from fruit and veggies likewise lack potassium, that mineral so essential to keeping our blood pressure low and our heart beating regularly. Potassium also supports our adrenal glands and our nervous system, making it a basic mineral for supporting our energy and our mood.

Perhaps most important, however, we need the fibre found in fruit, vegetables and whole grains to bind with toxins and expel them from our system. A low-carb diet is by definition a low-fibre diet. Ironically, low-carb diets increase our exposure to environmental toxins by eliminating the body's best defence, all in the name of reducing carb grams.

If this is bad for our health, it's worse for our weight. A clogged colon can cost you several kilograms as it loads up with impacted faecal matter. When you're not digesting food properly, you need to eat more to get the same nutrients and to feel 'full'.

These problems would be bad enough for people

remaining at their current weight. But dieters who lose up to 9 kg/20 lb in the first five months on a low-carb diet have virtually doubled their exposure to toxic material. Not only are they eating animal fats that are high in toxins but they are exposing themselves to these dangerous substances a second time when their own 'animal fat' melts away. Moreover, if they're suffering from the constipation and impaired elimination so common on these low-fibre programmes, they're attacked from a third quarter as well – the clogged, rotting faecal matter stuck within their own colons. The toxins are mounting, even as the fibre needed to help scrub these toxins away has been banned from their diets.

When I explained all of this to Mercedes, it was like a revelation. Her low-carb diet had put her at risk of symptoms that she'd never before experienced, so that even as she was losing weight she was also suffering from new problems. To add insult to injury, she had reached the point at which she had trouble losing weight or even maintaining the weight loss she'd already achieved.

Mercedes was luckier than she realised, though. There was one other common problem of low-carb diets that she had somehow managed to escape. My client Jewelle was not so lucky.

Low Stomach Acids: The X Factor in Low-Carb Diets

When Jewelle came to see me, she was nearly in tears.

'I don't understand why I'm having such a hard time

digesting my food,' she said. 'I used to be able to eat anything, and now I'm just gassy and uncomfortable every time I finish a meal. Plus' – she lowered her voice as though she were admitting something shameful – 'I have bad breath like you wouldn't believe. My boyfriend said something about it to me the other day, and I was so embarrassed! I don't understand why I'm having these problems.'

As I questioned Jewelle further, I found out what I had already begun to suspect. Jewelle had started a low-carb diet a few months earlier, an Atkins-style approach that involved eating lots of protein and very few fruit and vegetables. For her, the change was particularly dramatic, because she had been, as she put it, 'a real carb junkie' before she'd started the programme. Suddenly, instead of relying on pasta, bread and potatoes to fill her up, she'd switched to beef, chicken and cheese.

At first, she said, it felt wonderful. The high protein content of her diet had given her lots of energy, and she'd lost weight right away.

But then her troubles began. Gas, bloating and the bad breath she was so embarrassed about had set in, as well as severe heartburn after almost every meal. Although she'd taken some antacid tablets for the heartburn, they seemed to make her feel even worse.

'No wonder,' I told her. 'Your problem isn't too much stomach acid, but too little. All that protein on the low-carb diet, plus the lack of fruit and veggies, means that you're putting a huge strain on your stomach acid production without giving your system the vitamins and minerals it needs to make more stomach acid. I don't think your high-carb diet was so healthy, either, but at least it didn't put this kind of strain on your stomach.'

I suggested that Jewelle take some betaine hydrochloric acid (HC1) tablets supplemented with pepsin and bile extract to help restore her stomach acids. I also told her about the Fast Track. The Liver-Loving and Colon-Caring Foods in the Seven-Day Prequel would help provide the nutrients she was missing, I explained, while the *Fast Track Detox Diet* would begin an internal cleansing process, helping get rid of the toxins lurking in her meat and cheese. I pointed out that betaine HC1, pepsin and bile supplements are part of the Three-Day Sequel of my Fast Track, but that in her case, she might start taking them immediately.

Jewelle came to see me the week after she'd completed the Fast Track. She reported with relief that her symptoms had cleared up as soon as she'd begun taking the tablets. And the Seven-Day Prequel and Three-Day Sequel had given her a new appreciation of fruit and veggies.

'I feel like my entire body is breathing a huge sigh of relief,' she told me. 'I still want to lose weight – but not the low-carb way. It's just not worth it.'

Why You Must Prepare for Your Fast

In the middle of difficult lies opportunity.

– ALBERT EINSTEIN

My client Marcy was confused. I had just suggested that she try the Fast Track, both as a way to jump-start the weight loss she was looking for and to help purge her system of the toxins and pollutants that I could see were weighing her down.

Marcy was a lovely woman in her mid-twenties whose skin still showed traces of the acne that had plagued her throughout her adolescence. Although she'd been an energetic teenager, she felt that she was wearing herself out as an adult, working long hours as an associate at her law firm all week and then sleeping ten or even twelve hours every Saturday and Sunday. Disciplined and committed, Marcy tried to watch what she ate and make time for a regular workout routine, but she was discouraged by the sense that she was fighting a losing battle with both her weight and her energy level. I sensed she was also troubled by how much of her life was dominated by work and how little time she had for herself and the people she loved.

The *Fast Track Detox Diet*, I suggested, could clear her skin, restore her vitality, and help her rebalance both her hunger and her priorities. Marcy liked the sound of all that, but she couldn't quite get behind the idea of a day without food.

'I always heard that fasting was absolutely the worst way to lose weight,' she told me. 'Maybe you lose a little weight on that one day – if you can make it through! But then your metabolism is so messed up that you just gain it all back right away, and have an even harder time taking it off.'

Without proper nutritional support, that was true, I agreed. But that's the advantage of the Fast Track. You begin with a Seven-Day Prequel, fortifying your liver and stimulating your colon to eliminate waste properly by eating Liver-Loving and Colon-Caring Foods; drinking lots of pure water; and avoiding such Detox Detractors as alcohol, refined sugar, gluten, soya isolates, caffeine, the wrong kinds of fats and mould. On your One-Day Fast, you drink a delicious spiced juice made of cranberries and citrus, with ingredients carefully chosen to blunt your hunger, balance your blood sugar, rev up your metabolism and nourish your organs. Then a Three-Day Sequel helps ease you back into eating and ensures you get the fibre and water you need to rid your system of any remaining toxins. You seal in the results of your fast by consuming natural food sources of probiotics, which help restore the friendly bacteria you need to keep your digestive and immune systems working at optimum levels.

Marcy seemed sceptical until I told her that I myself have been using the One-Day Fast for the past year and a half – but only as part of an eating plan that includes a daily dose of Liver-Loving and Colon-Caring Foods. In fact, I explained, I use the One-Day Fast periodically to rid myself of the 'travel bloat' and toxic feeling I get from being in aeroplanes all the time.

'Think of this One-Day Fast as a purification for your body, mind and spirit,' I told her. 'But you're absolutely right – you can't just stop eating. You have to follow the protocol.'

Marcy still seemed uncertain about why, under some circumstances, a one-day fast could be a supremely healthy choice, while under other circumstances, it posed real dangers to your health, metabolism and weight-loss goals. I explained that the secret lies in understanding how your liver and colon work, so you can give them proper support.

Love Your Liver

After more than two decades working as a nutritionist, I'll admit it, I am in awe of the liver. As far as I'm concerned, this amazing organ nestled away in the right side of the abdomen has more than earned its name, which derives from an Old English word for 'life'. The liver is your key to life, even possessing the unique ability to regenerate itself. Although your liver may need up to two years for this regeneration process, you can rebuild this vital organ with the right diet and detox plan. The Seven-Day Prequel will help regenerate your liver with Liver-Loving Foods that will keep it running smoothly and promote its detoxification. But first, let's get to know a little more about your body's hardest-working organ.

A Living Filter

Your liver is your largest internal organ, responsible for a number of processes that help keep your body in balance. It regulates your blood flow, supports your digestive system and, if you're a woman, keeps your menstrual cycles running in peak condition.

One of your liver's most important functions, and the one most crucial to your weight loss, is breaking down everything that enters your body, from the healthiest bite of organic food to the poisonous pesticides that linger on your salad; from the purest filtered water to a glass of wine or a cup of coffee; from your daily vitamin and mineral supplements to the blood-pressure medication that your doctor has prescribed. It's your liver's job to distinguish between the nutrients you need to absorb and the toxins that must be filtered out of your bloodstream. By the way, medications, even if they're beneficial in other ways, are experienced as toxins by the liver, so if you're taking any kind of medication – prescription or otherwise – that's one more item that your liver has to filter out.

That's why, if you're asking your liver to do extra work, such as during the One-Day-Fast, it's *crucial* to give your liver heavy-duty nutritional support, supplying it with the Liver-Loving Foods it needs while protecting it from Detox Detractors. Otherwise, you could end your detox with a weaker system and an even more toxic liver than when you began. And because a poorly functioning liver contributes to weight gain and weight retention, an improperly done fast will leave you in worse shape than you were in before.

Caring for Your Colon

Your liver is your major detox organ. Like the oil filter for a car, it tries to remove the gunk and sludge from your system. Your colon, on the other hand, is your body's plumbing system. A high-functioning colon will efficiently expel waste from your body, keeping you healthy, symptom-free and ready to lose weight. But if your colon is clogged and toxic, as so many of our colons are, you're likely to encounter health problems as well as weight issues.

Ideally, food should remain in your system for only twelve to eighteen hours before your colon eliminates it as waste. Most British adults, however, retain waste for two to seven days – with disastrous results for their health. The longer those waste products sit in your colon, the more opportunity for toxins to penetrate back into your bloodstream, where your poor, overworked liver has to deal with them all over again. As a result, your body, especially your fat, becomes overloaded with toxic residues.

Unfortunately, the wrong kind of diet makes it more difficult for the colon to do its job. For example, your colon normally produces a certain amount of mucus to help move the faeces along. But when toxins, drugs, medication, stress or other factors irritate your colon, your organ protects itself by producing excess mucus. If you've been eating refined flour or sugar, its gluey, starchy residue binds with the excess mucus to create a layer of hardened faeces that builds up on your colon walls. The delicate little villi – waving hair-like stalks that line your colon and are designed to absorb nutrients and transport them into the bloodstream – become encased in this faecal layer. And the more your colon becomes encrusted with impacted faeces, the narrower the opening for your bowel movements. Between the hardened old faeces and the slow-moving new waste material, you've created a toxic breeding ground for bacteria and parasites.

Constipation is one possible result. And clearly, constipation is a big problem; millions of pounds are spent annually on laxatives, and doctors see thousands of patients each year concerned about this issue. But even if you're regular, or suffer from diarrhoea, you might still have a 'dirty colon'. And if you've been consuming lots of meat, chicken and dairy products (as is recommended on an Atkins-type low-carb diet), your colon is soon buried under a load of putrefying protein.

Many conventional doctors deny that faecal matter accumulates in this way and downplay the dangers of a toxic colon. But I look at the rise of colon-related illnesses, including Crohn's disease, diverticulitis, colitis and colon cancer, and draw what to me is an obvious conclusion: our clogged, toxic colons are putting us at risk.

It's not just bodily wastes that are festering in your colon, either. Heavy metals, pollutants and the remains of drugs and medication can stay behind with the other waste, releasing their toxins into the poisonous mixture.

You saw in Chapter 2 the kinds of symptoms that might result from a clogged or toxic colon. Even if you are symptom-free, however, a poorly functioning colon will weigh you down. You may literally be carrying extra weight in excess faecal matter, which from the outside looks like tummy fat, but which from the inside looks like faecal sludge or dried, encrusted faecal matter. Adding insult to injury, this encrustation keeps you from getting the most out of the food you eat, preventing your body from fully absorbing and assimilating nutrients. Many people notice that when their colons are cleansed, they can eat a third to a half of the amount they were used to before, yet feel even more satisfied, energised and nourished.

Ready, Set, Glow!

Marcy appreciated the mini science lesson I gave her, and she was happy to learn more about how the Fast Track would support her liver and her colon while she fasted. She also realised – as I hope you will, too – how important it was to support her liver and her colon *all* the time, not only when she was preparing for a fast. Armed with the dietary suggestions (discussed in the next chapter), she was ready both for her One-Day Fast and for the rest of her life.

> I work in a supermarket and was able to not be tempted by all the food. I go to work at 5 am. At 9 am I usually take a break and get something to eat. I started to get hungry then, but I kept drinking the cranberry water mixture and I got over that point of hunger. I noticed that my stomach went down in size, and I am not bloated. I like the thought of cleaning out my system. It sure worked for me – I lost weight and could see it on my own scales.
>
> – CINDY FICCARO, FORTY-SEVEN; LOST 1.8 KG/4 LB

CHAPTER

4

Getting Ready: The Seven-Day Prequel

*Before everything else,
getting ready is the secret of success.*

– HENRY FORD

THE FAST TRACK PREQUEL – 7 DAYS

Prepare for Your One-Day Fast with This Simple, Six-Step Programme

1. EACH DAY, CHOOSE AT LEAST ONE LIVER-LOVING FOOD FROM EACH GROUP BELOW: I'VE INCLUDED ENOUGH IDEAS HERE TO MAKE YOUR SEVEN-DAY PREQUEL SIMPLE, BUT IF YOU WANT MORE DETAILS OF FOOD OPTIONS FOR EACH GROUP, YOU'LL FIND THEM IN *THE FAST TRACK DETOX DIET*, PUBLISHED BY CENTURY.

1. The Crucifers (40 g/1½ oz cooked or an
   amount about the size of a small fist raw)
   cabbage, cauliflower, broccoli
2. Green Leafy Vegetables and Herbs (60 g/2 oz)
   parsley, kale, watercress, chard, coriander,
   beetroot, endive
3. Citrus (1 orange or the juice of ½ a lemon or
   lime)
   orange, lemon, lime
4. Sulphur-Rich Foods
   garlic (at least one clove, finely chopped),
   onions (60 g/2 oz cooked, about the size of a
   small fist), eggs (2)
5. Liver Healers
   artichoke (1 small artichoke or 4 cooked
   artichoke hearts), asparagus (5 medium spears
   cooked), beetroot (75 g/2½ oz cooked or raw),
   celery (2 medium sticks), dandelion root tea (1
   to 2 cups)

II. Each day, choose at least two of the
following Colon-Caring Foods:
   Milled or ground flaxseeds (2 to 3 tablespoons),
   carrot (1 small raw), apple (1 small raw with
   skin), pear (1 small raw with skin)

III. Each day, drink half your body weight in
ounces of filtered or purified water. (So, for
example, if you weigh 150 pounds you'll need to
drink 75 fluid ounces (4.7 pints) of water.)

IV. EACH DAY, MAKE SURE YOU HAVE AT LEAST TWO SERVINGS (THE SIZE OF THE PALM OF YOUR HAND) OF PROTEIN IN THE FORM OF LEAN BEEF, VEAL, LAMB, SKINLESS CHICKEN, TURKEY OR FISH, OR, IF YOU'RE A VEGAN OR VEGETARIAN, AT LEAST 2 TABLESPOONS A DAY OF A HIGH-QUALITY BLUE-GREEN ALGAE OR SPIRULINA SOURCE.

V. EACH DAY, MAKE SURE YOU HAVE 1 TO 2 TABLESPOONS OF OIL IN THE FORM OF OLIVE OIL, FLAXSEED, OR WOMAN'S OIL (A FLAXSEED OIL-BLACKCURRANT-SEED OIL BLEND)

VI. AVOID THE FOLLOWING DETOX DETRACTORS:

- *Excess fat*, especially trans fats from margarine and processed and fried foods
- *Sugar and all its relatives*, including high-fructose corn syrup, honey, molasses, sugar cane crystals, pure sugar cane juice, evaporated cane juice, dried cane juice, maltodextrin, and all products ending in '-ose' (such as sucrose, dextrose, fructose and levulose)
- *Artificial sweeteners*, including aspartame, sucralose or Splenda, and sugar alcohols (such as maltitol, mannitol, sorbitol and xylitol)
- *Refined carbohydrates*, including white rice and products made from white flour
- *Gluten*, found in wheat, rye, barley and all their

products (including bread, pasta, crackers), also found in many 'low-carb' products (such as packaged cereals, macaroni cheese, pizza-dough mix, spaghetti, shells, tortillas, pancake/waffle mixes and biscuits), and in vegetable proteins, modified food starch, some soy sauces and distilled vinegars.

- *Soya protein isolates*, found in low-carb 'energy' bars and soya protein powders, and processed soya foods (such as soya milk, soya cheese, soya ice cream, soya hot dogs and soya burgers)
- *Alcohol; over-the-counter drugs; and caffeine*, including coffee, tea, fizzy drinks and chocolate
- *Mould*, found on overly ripe fruits (especially melons, bananas and tropical fruits)

WARNING: If you do not follow the Prequel for the full seven days, please do not attempt the *Fast Track Detox Diet*. You might end up more bloated, constipated and 'toxic' than you were before, which could put a halt to your weight-loss efforts. Fasting without prior liver and colon support releases into your bloodstream the toxins that were previously lodged in your fat cells. These poisons can then relocate and settle in any number of organs, making you feel tired, anxious, headachy and more fatigued than when you started. You'll also be likely to gain more weight.

The Seven-Day Prequel:
Preparing for Detox

Now that you understand why supporting your liver and colon are so important, let's take a closer look at how the foods in the Seven-Day Prequel are intended to do just that.

STOCKING THE STAPLES:
YOUR SHOPPING LIST FOR THE FAST TRACK

- *Your choice of ten days' worth of crucifers:* cabbage, cauliflower, broccoli
- *Your choice of ten days' worth of green leafy vegetables:* parsley, kale, watercress, chard, coriander or beetroot
- *Your choice of ten days' worth of citrus:* oranges, lemons, limes, plus 2 oranges and 1 lemon to make the Miracle Juice
- *Your choice of ten days' worth of sulphur-rich foods:* garlic, onions, eggs
- *Your choice of ten days' worth of Liver-Loving Foods:* artichokes or artichoke hearts, asparagus, beetroot, dandelion root tea
- *Your choice of ten days' worth of Colon-Caring Foods:* milled or ground flaxseeds, carrots, apples, pears

- *Cranberry Juice:* 240 ml/8 fl oz of unsweetened cranberry juice or I jar unsweetened cranberry juice concentrate. Be sure to look for cranberry juice that has no sugar, corn syrup, or other juices added, including apple or grape
- *Spices:* fresh and non-irradiated cinnamon, ginger and nutmeg
- *3 days' worth of yoghurt or raw sauerkraut or I head of cabbage, mustard seeds and cumin and Maldon Sea Salt*
- 3 cups of fresh sprouts: mung bean, alfalfa, radish, broccoli, or lentil (store-bought or home-made)

* Ideally, your fruit and vegetables should be purchased on the day you plan to eat them.

If you have trouble finding any of these products at your local supermarket or health-food shop, or if you'd like to consider taking some supplements to boost your detox, see the complete *Fast Track Detox Diet.*

I. EACH DAY, CHOOSE AT LEAST ONE LIVER-LOVING FOOD FROM EACH GROUP

1. **The Crucifers (40 g/1½ oz cooked or raw, the size of a small fist)**
   cabbage, cauliflower, Brussels sprouts, broccoli, sprouting broccoli

Cruciferous veggies stimulate the phase 1 and phase 2 liver-detox pathways. Broccoli, cauliflower and cabbage enhance the process known as glutathione conjugation, in which the liver converts fat-soluble toxins into water-soluble substances that can be passed out through the urine.

Crucifers of all types also contain vital phyto-nutrients (nutrients found only in plants), such as indole-3-carbinol and sulphoraphane, which aid the liver in neutralising chemicals and drugs.

Remember how the two-phase liver-detox process creates so many free radicals? That means antioxidants are a crucial form of liver support, and crucifers are an excellent source of the antioxidant vitamin C.

2. **Green Leafy Vegetables and Herbs (60 g/2 oz)**
   parsley, kale, watercress, chard, coriander, beet-root

Chlorophyll-rich greens are powerful blood purifiers and natural internal deodorisers. They're also a great source of magnesium, one of the minerals that helps the liver manufacture enzymes smoothly and efficiently. Your body also needs magnesium for over 350 cellular processes – and all of your 650 muscles need it every second of every day. Magnesium is an anti-anxiety mineral, a major muscle relaxant and a natural laxative to boot.

The bitter taste of such greens as chard and kale stimulates digestive secretions. In Asian medicine, bitter-tasting foods are considered to be particularly healthy for the liver, perhaps because of the association between bitterness and bile.

Coriander is a savoury herb known in alternative medicine circles for its mercury-chelating properties. New research now suggests that coriander is also effective in eradicating salmonella, the nasty bacterium that can cause illness and even death.

3. Citrus (1 orange or juice of ½ fresh lemon or lime)
orange, lemon, lime

Oranges, lemons and limes are full of vitamin C, perhaps the most liver-loving vitamin of them all. Vitamin C stimulates the production of glutathione, the liver's premier antioxidant, which is crucial for a successful progression through the two-phase detox process. You can't take glutathione supplements by themselves because the molecules are too large to be absorbed by your gastrointestinal tract; so, if you want to be sure you've got enough of this vital antioxidant, load up on vitamin C. By stimulating glutathione, vitamin C also helps bind up heavy metals like mercury and cadmium and eliminate them from your body.

Vitamin C is also essential for acetylation, the process whereby the body eliminates potentially toxic sulpha drugs.

Tip: Squeeze lemon or lime juice into your daily dose of water, and try fresh lemon or lime juice to add some zing to your salads.

4. **Sulphur-Rich Foods**
   garlic (at least one clove, preferably raw), onions
   (60 g/2 oz finely chopped, cooked, about the size
   of a small fist), eggs (2)

One of the processes by which the liver eliminates
toxins is known as *sulphation* – so called because sulphur
is an indispensable part of the procedure. These
sulphur-rich foods make toxins easier to eliminate.

Eggs are rich in the amino acids methionine,
cysteine, glycine, glutamine and taurine. As we've seen,
your liver needs these acids (also found in whey) to
successfully complete phase 2 of its detox process. And
eggs offer the cholesterol your liver needs to produce
that beautiful bile.

5. **Liver Healers**
   artichoke (1 small or 4 cooked hearts), asparagus
   (5 medium spears, cooked), beetroot (75 g/2½ oz
   cooked or raw), dandelion root tea (1 to 2 cups)

Artichokes, especially the hearts, contain powerful
antioxidants known as flavonoids that protect the liver's
cells and tissues. Artichokes are also good for the
secretion of bile, which, as we've seen, helps the body
better digest and assimilate fats. The artichoke is a close
relative of milk thistle, queen of the liver protectors,
which offers major defence against free radicals and is
especially good for people with compromised immunity
or alcohol-related liver problems. If you're looking for

more artichoke in your diet, you'll love Absolutely Artichoke Soup which you'll find in Chapter 8.

Asparagus contains high amounts of vitamin A and potassium, another mineral on which the liver depends during detox.

Beetroot is full of betaine, which helps protect the liver against the damaging effects of alcohol. Betaine also thins the bile and helps it move freely within the bile ducts.

Dandelion root stimulates liver function. It also contains inulin, a fibre-like substance that functions as a *probiotic* – an element that helps nourish the friendly bacteria in the gut. As if that weren't enough, the humble dandelion root is also good for lowering the blood sugar.

VARIETY IS THE SPICE OF LIFE

I wanted to keep this Seven-Day Prequel as simple as possible, so I've given you lots of leeway to choose the foods you like and find easy to prepare. But I also want to urge you to vary your food choices as much as you can, and you can find more suggestions in the complete, unabridged book. There's still a lot we don't yet know about nutrition, especially when it comes to the exciting new field of phytonutrients, which have remarkable healing benefits, warding off disease and promoting optimal health. The more different kinds of fruit and vegetables you eat, the greater your chance of getting the full benefit of all of Nature's phytonutrients. Still, if you find yourself eating the same green leafy vegetable seven days in a row, don't worry. The main thing is to eat one item from each Liver-Loving Food category. Enjoy!

II. EACH DAY, CHOOSE AT LEAST TWO OF THE
FOLLOWING COLON-CARING FOODS
milled or ground flaxseeds (2 to 3 tablespoons), carrot (1 small raw), apple (1 small raw with skin), pear (1 small raw with skin)

Flaxseeds are a two-for-one fibre source, because they contain both soluble and insoluble fibre, as well as lignans — oestrogen-modulating substances that have antiviral, antibacterial and antifungal properties. Because of their effect on oestrogen, flaxseeds are especially helpful for women suffering from PMS, perimenopause and menopausal challenges.

I like Fibro Flax, which is just flaxseeds, but I'm also quite fond of Men's Fibro Flax, a combination of fibre sources made from cold-milled certified organic flaxseeds, pumpkin-seed meal and zinc sulphate. Produced by the company Health from the Sun, the organic flaxseeds it contains are further purified by an infra-red lamp that kills mycotoxins (mould-containing elements) on the seed. See Detox Detractors, below, for more on the dangers of mould. *Women take note:* ignore the name and treat yourself to a zinc-rich source of fibre made from an organic source and already ground up for your convenience.

Tip: Fibro Flax and Men's Fibro Flax add a delicious, nutty taste when stirred into smoothies, yoghurt or cottage cheese and when sprinkled over salads.

The fruit and veggies I've recommended are not only a wonderful source of fibre but also a terrific way to up your vitamin C intake and your antioxidant quotient. You'll find these delicious foods filling, as well, a good way to put your hunger to rest while giving your taste buds a treat.

IF YOU DON'T NEED TO LOSE WEIGHT OR IF YOU ARE PRONE TO DEPRESSION (SEROTONIN DEFICIENT), YOU CAN ALSO CHOOSE FROM THESE SOURCES OF FIBRE:

- *Nuts and seeds:* One serving would be a handful of almonds, walnuts, or sunflower seeds. Eat them raw or toast them yourself at home, but don't buy oven-roasted products, which are more likely to contain additives.
- *Friendly carbs:* A single serving is 90 g/3 oz of chickpeas, lentils, adzuki beans, kidney beans or 170 g/6 oz of oatmeal or 1 small sweet potato.

III. EACH DAY, DRINK HALF YOUR BODY WEIGHT IN OUNCES OF FILTERED OR PURIFIED WATER

The many amazing health benefits from plain old H_2O are too numerous for me to go into here. I'll just restrict myself to explaining how water helps detoxify your system by carrying out waste products more efficiently and helping your liver, colon and digestive system to do their jobs. Your blood is 83 per cent water, and it needs a good volume of water to help it carry the toxins and waste products that we've known travel through it and to transport the nutrients it carries to every part of our body. Our cells, too, need water to carry away their metabolic waste products. And, of course, our colons need water to help with the crucial task of eliminating waste.

Throughout my years of nutritional counselling, I've been struck by how many of my clients have told me they've felt hungry when I could tell, from their symptoms and eating habits, that they were really thirsty. Try drinking a few glasses of water at least twenty minutes before a meal and see if you don't require less food to feel full. Notice, too, the refreshed, energised feeling that drinking lots of water will give you.

When you do drink, remember that water is best taken at room temperature between meals, though you can drink up to a half a glass of water (120 ml/4 fl oz) during meals. Drinking too much of *any* liquid while eating can dilute your hydrochloric acid, which is so necessary in the digestion of protein and the assimilation of acid-based minerals such as calcium and iron. And wait until two hours after you've eaten to drink any more.

Most of us tend to be dehydrated, drinking too little water and too much coffee, tea and caffeinated fizzy drinks. These all tend to dry us out, thanks to the diuretic properties of caffeine. If you wait to drink until you're actually thirsty, you've waited too long: dehydration starts long before we're conscious of it. So make sure you drink at least half your body weight in ounces throughout your day. And don't substitute another fluid, particularly during the entire time you are on the Fast Track. It's *water* that your body needs. You may be surprised at how much better you feel when this need is finally met.

IV. EACH DAY, MAKE SURE YOU HAVE AT LEAST TWO
SERVINGS (THE SIZE OF THE PALM OF YOUR HAND)
OF PROTEIN IN THE FORM OF LEAN ORGANIC BEEF,
VEAL, LAMB, SKINLESS CHICKEN, TURKEY OR FISH OR,
IF YOU'RE A VEGAN OR VEGETARIAN, AT LEAST 2
TABLESPOONS A DAY OF A HIGH-QUALITY BLUE-
GREEN ALGAE OR SPIRULINA SOURCE

You already know you need protein for energy, muscle building and many other vital functions – but did you know that protein is also crucial to the detox process? Protein activates the production of the enzymes that your detox system needs to break down toxins into water-soluble substances so they can be eliminated from the body. So when you're preparing for your Seven-Day Prequel, don't forget the protein!

WATER, WATER, EVERYWHERE . . .

I wouldn't tell you to avoid bottled water, if only because I want to make this Seven-Day Prequel as easy as I can for you. But you should be aware that quality-control standards for bottled water are often less rigorous than those for tap water. 'Mineral' waters are tested for thirteen chemicals and bacteria – less than a quarter as many substances as tap water. There are also no requirements, as there are for tap water, for mineral waters to be tested daily or even weekly. For 'spring' waters, there is no legislation at all.

So if you're really concerned about high-quality H_2O, your best bet is a home filtration system.

V. Each day, make sure you have 1 to 2 tablespoons of oil in the form of olive oil, flaxseed oil or Woman's Oil (a flaxseed oil-blackcurrant-seed oil blend)

You need oil to lubricate your intestines, helping your colon more easily pass all waste products – and the toxins they carry – out of your body. Flaxseed oil and Woman's Oil will also provide you with a healthy source of the fat-burning omega-3s, to aid in weight loss as well as detox. The Woman's Oil contains blackcurrant-seed oil, a source of the 'good' omega-6 fatty acids, which is also a natural weight-loss aid and terrific for beautiful skin.

VI. Avoid the following Detox Detractors

- excess fat, especially trans fats from margarine and processed and fried foods
- sugar and all its relatives, including high-fructose corn syrup, honey, molasses, sugar cane crystals, pure sugar cane juice, evaporated cane juice, dried cane juice, maltodextrin, and all products ending in '-ose' (such as sucrose, dextrose, fructose and levulose)
- artificial sweeteners, including aspartame, sucralose or Splenda, and sugar alcohols (such as maltitol, mannitol, sorbitol and xylitol)
- refined carbohydrates, including white rice and products made from white flour
- gluten, found in wheat, rye, barley and all their products (including bread, pasta, crackers), also found in many 'low-carb' products (such as packaged cereals, macaroni cheese, pizza dough mix, spaghetti, shells, tortillas, pancake/waffle mixes and biscuits) and in vegetable proteins, modified food starch, some soy sauces and distilled vinegars
- soya protein isolates, found in low-carb 'energy'

bars and soya protein powders, and processed
soya foods (such as soya milk, soya cheese, soya ice
cream, soya hot dogs and soya burgers)
- alcohol; over-the-counter drugs; and caffeine,
including coffee, tea, fizzy drinks and chocolate
- mould, found on overly ripe fruits (especially
melons, bananas and tropical fruits)

These Detox Detractors either lower enzyme activity
during phases 1 and 2 detox, interrupting the liver's
efforts to transform toxins into non-toxic metabolites,
or are linked to a decreased absorption of necessary
detox nutrients. Therefore you must avoid them during
the seven days before your fast, or you'll start your fast
with an increased toxic load. Given this extra burden,
your liver will be slowed down in its efforts to
metabolise fat and detoxify your body, which will both
impede your weight-loss efforts and leave you feeling
sluggish, weak and low on energy. Here's a closer look at
how each Detox Detractor works its evil magic.

Excess fat, especially trans fat, strains both your liver
and your colon, so, during the Seven-Day Prequel,
avoid foods that are processed, refined or fried, such as
many biscuits, sweets, cakes and crackers. You might
even cut back on the 'good fat' foods at this time –
peanut butter and almond butter; excessive nuts, such as
almonds, peanuts and cashews; seeds; avocados; and
even salad dressings, including the very best virgin olive
oil, coconut oil or macadamia nut oil. Any of these
otherwise healthy fats can be hard for the liver to break

down if your bile is congested or thickened with toxins. And, of course, trans fats are dangerous at all times, so stay away from processed vegetable oils, margarine, vegetable shortenings and baked goods made from these oils. As of 1 January 2006, US food labels will have to list trans fat content. However, there are currently no such plans to do so on UK labels.

Sugar and other sweeteners, natural or artificial, stress both your liver and your colon. Moreover, both natural sugar and sugar alcohols have the potential to feed yeast, a known liver stressor because of the aldehydes that are formed – substances that overload the detox pathways and inhibit the action of the detox enzymes.

Refined carbohydrates, along with sugar, are deadly to both detox and weight loss. Not only do they inhibit the liver's detox pathways, but they create those roller-coaster highs and lows in blood sugar, insulin, hunger and cravings. Due to these blood sugar and insulin ups and downs the white stuff – whether sugar, flour or white rice – is most likely to be stored as fat.

Gluten, as we've seen, is one of the big hidden dangers in low-carb diet products. As its name suggests, it creates a gluey substance that can bind with fat and mucus to cover the intestinal villi and clog your colon, which is particularly dangerous for those who have been on a low-fibre diet like Atkins (or like the typical British diet). Gluten intolerance is more prevalent than previously recognised, so don't tempt trouble; during your Seven-Day Prequel, avoid low-carb products made with gluten as well as bread, wheat, rice and other gluten-bearing grains.

Soya protein isolates are incomplete proteins that lack the sulphur-bearing amino acids methionine and cysteine. The high-phytic acid in unfermented and processed soya products disrupt mineral absorption and can deplete your supply of zinc, magnesium and calcium, which you need for liver detox. (Miso and tempe, which are forms of fermented soya, are fine.)

Alcohol, drugs and caffeine are liver stressors that tax the detox pathways big time. So definitely axe the alcohol, soft drinks and colas – and avoid both regular and decaffeinated coffee as well as black and green tea.

Sadly, green tea is a no-no because an increasing body of studies has shown that it is contaminated with aluminium fluoride from pesticides and fertilisers. Fluoride cues your organs, including your liver and your brain, to stockpile aluminium, with sometimes disastrous results. Fluoride is also a known thyroid suppressor. With an estimated 10 to 25 per cent of the UK population suffering from hypothyroidism, and considering all the fluoride you're consuming in your water, toothpaste, soft drinks and foods processed with fluoridated water, do you really want to take a chance of 'fluoridated' green tea? Recent samples of green tea were also found to contain the pesticides DDT and its cousin, the DDT-like Dursban. Although DDT has been banned in the United States since 1972 and in Britain since 1986, it can still find its way back to these countries from China or India in your tea bag. (If you really miss your tea, try a caffeine-free herbal blend, made from lemon, ginger, cinnamon, cloves or cranberry.

THE CAFFEINE CONNECTION

One of the hardest substances in the world to give up is caffeine, whether in the form of coffee, black or green tea, colas or chocolate. If you're used to a daily dose of caffeine, you may experience some withdrawal symptoms, such as headache, cravings, irritability, fatigue, depression, anxiety, nervousness, inability to concentrate, nausea, a runny nose and sudden fluctuations in body temperature.

All the Liver-Loving fruit and veggies you're consuming will up the vitamin C in your diet, sustaining your adrenal glands – those major stress glands that bear the brunt of caffeine highs and lows. They'll also combat withdrawal symptoms to some extent. Meanwhile, drinking half your body weight in ounces of water will help you flush the caffeine from your system. You can also try taking the Adrenal Formula, a glandular tissue extract that supports the adrenals and contains tyrosine, which seems to be helpful in curbing detox withdrawal systems.

However you do it, I strongly urge you to kick the caffeine habit before your One-Day Fast. Fast Trackers who gave up food and coffee at the same time ended up with caffeine headaches, mood

crashes, mental fog and fatigue on their fasting days.
Ease your transition into a caffeine-free day by using
this week to prepare.

Finally, avoid any unnecessary over-the-counter
drugs at this time (but don't stop taking prescription
medicines without consulting your doctor).

Mould can stress your liver, so avoid all sources of
mould, especially mouldy fruit, because some fruit
moulds produce mycotoxins that can cause severe liver
damage, cancer, breathing problems or allergic reactions.
Since fresh fruit is more susceptible to mould, consider
purchasing your fruit frozen. Remember to refrigerate
cut fresh fruit within two hours after serving, and don't
buy more fruit than you can use within a short time.
Inspect your fruit closely for signs of moulds or bruises,
particularly melons, peaches and nectarines, which are
especially susceptible.

TOO BUSY FOR VEGGIES?
AN ALTERNATIVE SEVEN-DAY PREQUEL

It's always best to support your liver and colon with real, whole foods. But if you're on your own fast track and know you won't be able to follow the protocols in this chapter, there is an alternative. For your convenience, supplements are available, and you can find more information about them in the complete *Fast Track Detox Diet*.

YOUR FAST TRACKER LOG: THE PREQUEL

DAY ONE

I. The Liver-Loving Foods I ate today
From Group 1: The Crucifers (40 g/1½ oz)
cabbage, cauliflower, broccoli

I. _____

Others: _____

From Group 2: Green Leafy Vegetables and Herbs (60 g/2 oz)
parsley, kale, watercress, chard, coriander, beetroot tops

I. _____

Others: _____

From Group 3: Citrus – each day, I orange or half the juice of a fresh lemon or lime
orange, lemon, lime

I. _____

Others: _____

From Group 4: Sulphur-Rich Foods – at least one serving daily of one of the following:
garlic (at least one clove, minced), onions (½ cup cooked – about the size of a small fist), eggs (2)

I. _____

Others: _____

From Group 5: Liver Healers – at least one serving daily of one of the following:
artichoke (I small artichoke or 4 cooked artichoke hearts), asparagus (5 medium spears cooked), beet-root (75 g/2½ oz cooked or I cup raw), dandelion root tea (I or 2 cups)

I. _____

Others: _____

II. The Colon-Caring Foods I ate today
milled or ground flaxseeds (2 to 3 tablespoons), carrot (I small raw), apple (I small raw with skin), pear (I small raw with skin), berries (125 g/4½ oz)

I. _____

2. _____

Others: _____

III. The water I drank today
Today I drank_____ml/fl oz of water.

IV. The oil I ate today
Today I consumed_____tablespoons of healthy oil.

V. Today I did/did not avoid all Detox Detractors.

My evaluation
How do I feel about how I stuck to the Fast Track today?

_____

_____

_____

What strategies worked for me?

_____

_____

_____

What will I do differently tomorrow?

_____

_____

_____

Duplicate this log and use it for each of your
Seven-Day Prequel.

The One-Day Fast

What would life be like if we had
no courage to attempt anything?

– VINCENT VAN GOGH

WARNING

Although fasting is an excellent link to better health for most people, there are some times in your life when you should not fast.

You should not fast if you are pregnant, nursing, recovering from an illness or injury, debilitated or malnourished, including those of you with aids, severe anaemia, wasting states or cancer. People with weakened immunity should not fast.

You should *not* fast if you have cardiac arrhythmia, type I diabetes, congestive heart failure, ulcers, liver disease or kidney disease, or if you are struggling with mental illness (including anxiety, depression, bipolar disorder or schizophrenia), as your condition may worsen if you fast.

You should *not* fast before or after surgery, as it might compromise your ability to heal.

You should *not* fast if you are more than 4.5 kg/10 lb underweight or if you are prone to eating disorders.

You should *consult your doctor and obtain permission to fast* if you are diabetic, hypoglycaemic or prone to severe migraines. Likewise, *consult your doctor* if you are taking regular medications, including antidepressants, blood-pressure medications and birth-control pills.

Recently, I had the opportunity to talk with three dieters who were about to embark on the One-Day-Fast portion of the *Fast Track Detox Diet*.

Lucy was a marketing analyst in her mid-twenties. A warm, exuberant woman who had struggled with her weight since before she was a teenager, she told me that even the Seven-Day Prequel had been difficult for her to maintain. Her old pattern had been to use coffee as an appetite suppressant, drinking a few cups throughout the morning to enable her to skip breakfast and eat a light lunch. Then she would 'reward' herself with a big dinner.

'I lost weight just on the Seven-Day Prequel,' she reported, 'and although I'm still a bit groggy from giving up coffee, I did like eating all those fruit and vegetables. But a whole day without food? It makes me kind of nervous. I'm afraid I'll be hungry all the time.'

Nila, a quiet, reserved woman in her mid-forties, had just returned to full-time work as a nurse after working part-time and raising her children for the past ten years. 'I often feel that I'm too busy to eat,' she told me. 'But my job is quite stressful and, on my days off, I have so many errands. I am concerned that if I eat nothing at all, I may simply collapse!'

Jason, a computer analyst in his early thirties, had been on my Fat Flush plan for nearly a year. He was pleased with how much weight he'd lost and how he'd been able to keep the weight off. Every so often, however, he'd indulge in a high-fat meal or a rich dessert, and given his sluggish metabolism, the weight showed up immediately. For him, the One-Day Fast was a kind of insurance policy, something he knew he could rely on if his weight began to creep up. Still, he admitted, he was used to a hearty breakfast, a good-sized lunch and frequent healthy snacks throughout the day. 'I have this image of getting weaker and weaker, until by the end of the day, I'm just lying on the sofa,' he admitted. 'I'd like to lose extra weight – and I'd sure like to know that I can always take off any extra weight. But how hard is it going to be?'

I was happy to reassure all three dieters that I'd specially designed the One-Day Fast to address just these concerns. The Fast Track Miracle Juice, a delicious blend of cranberry and citrus juices spiced with cinnamon, ginger and nutmeg, is composed of ingredients that staves off hunger, balances blood sugar and revs up metabolism.

I told these budding Fast Trackers of Anastasia Signoretta's experience, a twenty-seven-year-old Fast Tracker: 'I did it on the weekend, when I normally sit around and watch TV,' she reported. 'Instead, I cleaned my whole apartment' – and lost 1.6 kg/3½ lb. Of course, fasters should avoid strenuous exercise, but I did recommend a brisk twenty-minute walk or session on a rebounder (a mini trampoline), to help keep their lymph flowing and their blood moving. And I shared with them my own experience during one-day fasts, which always leaves me feeling lighter, cleaner and more energised.

Still, these three clients were a bit sceptical – until the day after the fast. Then they were all smiles. 'I wasn't even hungry!' Lucy said triumphantly. 'And by the end of the afternoon, I started to feel really good, like I'd somehow got free of something.'

'I had a little dip in energy around 2 pm,' Nila admitted. 'But I drank some more juice, and a glass of water, and slowly, I felt my energy flowing back. I ended up feeling calmer, more peaceful and more focused. It was a very interesting experience.'

'Hey, I felt like Superman,' Jason remarked. 'I don't know what it was, but I felt *strong*.'

THE FAST TRACK DETOX DIET MIRACLE JUICE PROTOCOL

To conduct your one-day fast, follow this simple, four-step programme:

1. PREPARE THE FOLLOWING 'MIRACLE JUICE'

1.8 litres/3¼ pints Cranberry Water
(recipe follows)
½ teaspoon ground cinnamon
¼ teaspoon ground ginger
¼ teaspoon ground nutmeg
180 ml/6 fl oz freshly squeezed orange juice
60 ml/2 fl oz freshly squeezed lemon juice
1 teaspoon 100% maple syrup to taste

1. Bring the Cranberry Water to a light boil; reduce the heat to low.
2. Place the cinnamon, ginger and nutmeg into a tea infuser; add to the Cranberry Water. (For a tangier juice, add the spices directly to the liquid.)
3. Simmer for 15 to 20 minutes; cool to room temperature.
4. Stir in the orange and lemon juices. Add maple syrup at this time, if desired.

Cranberry Water Recipe

To make 1.8 litres/3¼ pints, add 240 ml/8 fl oz unsweetened cranberry juice to 1.55 litres/2¾ pints filtered water OR 3 tablespoons unsweetened cranberry juice concentrate to 1.7 litres/3 pints of filtered water.

Be sure to look for cranberry juice that has no sugar, corn syrup or other juices added, including apple or grape.

II. ALTERNATE DRINKING ONE CUP (240 ML/8 FL OZ) OF FILTERED WATER AND ONE CUP (240 ML/8 FL OZ) OF MIRACLE JUICE DURING THE DAY. DRINK AT LEAST 2 LITRES/3½ PINTS OF FILTERED WATER THROUGHOUT THE DAY, IN ADDITION TO THE MIRACLE JUICE. MAKE SURE YOU DRINK AT LEAST A CUP OF LIQUID – EITHER THE MIRACLE JUICE OR WATER – EVERY HOUR.

Begin the protocol when you wake up in the morning. A sample day is provided below. You don't have to begin at a specific time, but be sure to have all eight glasses of Miracle Juice in addition to the 2 litres/3½ pints of water.

6 am	240 ml/8 fl oz	filtered water
7 am	240 ml/8 fl oz	Miracle Juice
8 am	240 ml/8 fl oz	filtered water
9 am	240 ml/8 fl oz	Miracle Juice
10 am	240 ml/8 fl oz	filtered water
11 am	240 ml/8 fl oz	Miracle Juice
12 pm	240 ml/8 fl oz	filtered water
1 pm	350 ml/12 fl oz	Miracle Juice
2 pm	240 ml/8 fl oz	filtered water
3 pm	240 ml/8 fl oz	Miracle Juice

4 pm	240 ml/8 fl oz	filtered water
5 pm	350 ml/12 fl oz	Miracle Juice
6 pm	240 ml/8 fl oz	filtered water
7 pm	240 ml/8 fl oz	Miracle Juice
8 pm	240 ml/8 fl oz	filtered water
9 pm	240 ml/8 fl oz	Miracle Juice
10 pm	240 ml/8 fl oz	filtered water

III. UPON RISING AND AT THE END OF THE DAY TAKE 1 SERVING OF A COLON-CARING SUPPLEMENT, CHOSEN FROM AMONG THE FOLLOWING:

- Powdered psyllium husks (1 to 2 teaspoons mixed in 240 ml/8 fl oz of water or Miracle Juice)
- Ground or milled flaxseeds (2 to 3 tablespoons mixed in 300 to 350 ml/10 to 12 fl oz of water or 240 ml/8 fl oz Miracle Juice)
- Super GI Cleanse (3 capsules, taken with 300 to 350 ml/10 to 12 fl oz of water or 240 ml/8 fl oz Miracle Juice.

IV. ENGAGE ONLY IN LIGHT EXERCISE – EITHER A 20-MINUTE WALK OR 10 MINUTES ON THE REBOUNDER.

(For more on exercise and fitness, see the *Fat Flush Fitness Plan* that I wrote with exercise guru Joannie Greggains.)

I was so pleased that these three Fast Trackers had such a good experience, though I'll admit I wasn't surprised. Healthy fasting – the kind supported by adequate nutritional preparation for the liver and sufficient fibre for the colon – is probably the best-kept secret I know to good health, long-term weight loss and an overall feeling of well-being. I was thrilled that my three Fast Trackers could share in this wonderful practice, and I'm even more thrilled to be sharing it with you.

So let's get started. Here's the protocol you should follow for your One-Day Fast, followed by an explanation of each element you'll consume and some idea of what you might expect during detox.

A Closer Look at the One-Day Fast

Every ingredient of the One-Day Fast has been specially chosen to stave off hunger; balance your blood sugar; rev up your metabolism; and keep you feeling fit, energised and trim throughout your fasting day.

The combination of cranberry and citrus juices in the brew is rich in vitamin C, or ascorbic acid. Among its many benefits, ascorbic acid thins and decongests the bile, making it easier for the liver to emulsify (break down) fat at peak efficiency. This combination is also very refreshing and 'cleansing' to the palate, offering a satisfying experience that helps mitigate against hunger pangs.

The orange and lemon juices, as we've seen in the Seven-Day Prequel, are key Liver-Loving Foods. Their vitamin C also stimulates the production of glutathione, the major antioxidant on which the liver relies to progress through its two-phase detox process. Vitamin C also helps bind heavy metals and eliminate potentially toxic sulpha drugs.

The *cranberry juice* helps flush away toxic fluids, which can account for as much as 4.5 to 6.8 kg/10 to 15 lb of water weight trapped in our tissues. This is the water weight that makes us look bloated; it literally weighs us down. Arbutin, a key ingredient in cranberries, is a diuretic that draws both toxins and fluids from our system.

Cranberries are rich in vitamins A, B_1, B_2, B_3, B_5, B_6, C and E, as well as in folic acid, boron, calcium, chromium, copper, iron, magnesium, manganese, molybdenum, phosphorus, potassium, selenium, sodium and sulphur, all crucial vitamins and minerals for liver activity, as well as for many other bodily functions. These potent red berries are also vital aids to liver detox because they contain exceedingly high levels of life-saving antioxidants that provide crucial support for both phase 1 and phase 2 detox pathways. Furthermore, their high content of organic acids – such as benzoic, malic, quinic, citric and ellagic acids – have outstanding therapeutic qualities for many bodily functions. Malic acid, for example, is a potent digestion regulator and helps protect against diarrhoea, while ellagic acid has been proven to inhibit the initiation of cancer.

The aromatic spices cinnamon, nutmeg and ginger all help rev up your metabolism and fight hunger.

Several years ago, a research team under the guidance of Dr Richard Anderson discovered that cinnamon contains a flavonoid compound that mimics the body's insulin-regulating activity to control blood sugar metabolism. This is good news, not just for people with type 2 diabetes but also for Fast Trackers. Overproduction of insulin causes your blood sugar to drop quickly, inducing hunger, whereas insulin itself encourages your body to store fat. So cinnamon's natural insulin-like properties will help keep your blood sugar level throughout the One-Day Fast, which in turn will work to reduce your hunger and cravings. Some researchers even believe that cinnamon is promising as a means of preventing type 2 diabetes.

THE AMAZING CRANBERRY

Cranberries have so many remarkable benefits, it's hard to know where to start. Since I first began studying this miracle fruit, a host of new cran benefits have come to light. Here's a quick tour:

- Preliminary research suggests that cranberries may be crucial ingredients in cancer prevention. Some researchers believe that cranberries interact positively with two enzymes that either create cancerous cells or help them proliferate. Others have found that cranberries contain elements that may inhibit the growth of colon or prostate cancer cells by protecting our DNA. Still other researchers believe that the quercitin in cranberries may help prevent breast and colon cancer that results from chemicals or toxins or might inhibit the growth of breast-cancer cells.

- New research suggests that elements in cranberries may help prevent atherosclerosis – the build-up of cholesterol, fat and plaque in the arteries – which is a leading contributor to cardiovascular disease. Scientists have theorised that atherosclerosis begins when low-density lipoprotein (LDL), which you've heard called the 'bad' cholesterol, becomes oxidised (affected by oxygen), creating an inflammatory response. This inflammation sets of a chain of events that might lead to arterial lesions and, ultimately, restricted blood flow. Cranberries, however, contain powerful antioxidants that seem to be able to prevent and even reverse this process.

- By the same token, cranberry juice may help raise high-density lipoprotein (HDL), or the 'good' cholesterol, according to research presented at the American Chemical Society's annual meeting in April 2004. Dr Joseph Vinson of the University of Scranton (Pennsylvania) conducted a study suggesting that drinking three glasses of cranberry juice a day might reduce heart disease by 40 per cent.

- Although research is still preliminary, some scientists are beginning to explore the possibility that cranberries can help prevent the formation of blood clots and even strokes. Some animal studies also suggest that cranberries can help decrease our body's LDL cholesterol.

- Early research suggests that cranberries might help prevent the formation of ulcers and other gastrointestinal diseases, primarily by inhibiting *Helicobacter pylori*, the bacteria that is implicated in many instances of ulcers and gastrointestinal conditions.

- South African researchers have conducted studies suggesting that cranberry juice may be helpful in preventing kidney stones.

- Cranberries seemed to help experimental subjects resist the effects of *E. coli* bacteria, and so to protect against urinary tract infection. Researchers were especially interested in cranberries' effectiveness against strains of *E. coli* that were resistant to antibiotics.

- Gum disease – the gateway to many other infections – also seems to respond well to the humble cranberry. Dental plaque is a breeding ground for bacteria and other micro-organisms that can serve as precursors to a wide range of diseases, including caries (cavities) and periodontal conditions. Cranberry in various forms seems able to help experimental subjects clear the bacteria from their mouths.

- Among the most potent elements in cranberries are polyphenols, a kind of plant-based anti-oxidant that has powerful health-inducing effects. Laboratory studies have shown that 240 ml/8 fl oz of cranberry juice contain 567 milligrams of polyphenols – compared to 0.53 milligrams in apple juice and 400 milligrams in red wine. Just 60 ml/2 fl oz of fresh cranberries contain 373 milligrams of polyphenols, more than much larger servings of oranges, broccoli, blueberries, strawberries, bananas, apples or white grapes.

The warming effects of nutmeg make this spice an aid to digestion, reducing flatulence and helping fight hunger and combat cravings. You may also be interested to know that nutmeg is a powerful aphrodisiac.

Ginger is a peppery and pungent natural vasodilator – a substance that causes the blood vessels to expand. As blood flows more freely through the expanded vessels, your body heat rises and your metabolism revs up along with it. According to an Australian study published in the *International Journal of Obesity*, ginger can cause a metabolic boost of as much as 20 per cent, an effect that Anastasia clearly felt when she used her fast day to clean her apartment instead of watching TV as she usually did.

FRESH IS BEST!

Have you ever noticed the way spices tend to pile up in your kitchen for months, sometimes years at a time? It happens to all of us – but the problem is that kept in this way, spices tend to lose their potency. If you've stored them over the stove, the heat sucks away their therapeutic value; if you keep them in the fridge or the freezer, they dry out too quickly. Either way, their health-giving properties evaporate along with their flavour, and much of their benefit is lost.

So for the Miracle Juice, I want you to buy a fresh jar of each spice. Try to find organic and non-irradiated spices. On this detox day, you definitely don't want to add any additional toxins to your body!

Water, of course, helps flush the toxins from our system. It's always important to keep our bodies well hydrated, but it's super-important to do so during a fast. Drinking at least 2 litres/3½ pints of pure, filtered water along with the juice will keep you feeling refreshed and 'full', even as it helps carry the toxins out of your system.

Colon-Caring fibre – whether in the form of psyllium, flaxseed or Super GI-Cleanse – is the final crucial element of your One-Day Fast. As we've seen, fibre helps scrub your colon clean, breaking down any clogged or impacted faecal matter that might be clinging to your colon walls and ensuring that you won't become constipated or bloated when you resume eating. Fibre also binds with the toxins released during your fast. Think of all the pollutants, additives and other poisons that might be stored in the 1.4 to 3.6 kg/3 to 8 lb of fat you're going to release on your fasting day, and then make sure you ingest enough fibre to soak them up.

TO WEIGH OR NOT TO WEIGH?

I strongly urge you to weigh yourself only twice during this part of the Fast Track – once on the morning you begin the One-Day Fast, and once at the same time on the following morning. As the day proceeds, you may be tempted to run to the scales and see how it's going – but resist that temptation! Losing weight, particularly as measured in kilograms or pounds, is not a linear process; it proceeds in an irregular fashion, with sudden drops and occasionally even unexplained increases as your body adjusts to this new regime. Find out your baseline when you begin the One-Day Fast, and then wait until the next morning to see how you *really* did. Any other numbers that show up along the way will only distort the situation.

Detox Symptoms: Positive and Negative

For most of my Fast Trackers, detox was an extremely positive experience. But for some, particularly those who felt themselves to be dependent on caffeinated drinks, the initial experience of the One-Day Fast was somewhat uncomfortable. Although many participants reported increased energy, mental clarity and well-being, some did experience other symptoms, including headaches, fatigue, irritability, foggy thinking and mild depression.

The explanation is simple: having stored the toxins in our fat, we pay a price for getting rid of them. As we burn up stored body fat for fuel, the oil-soluble toxins we've stored in our fat are also released, sometimes causing distress as they recirculate through the system. If you've been diligent about following the Seven-Day Prequel, and particularly if you've been following the Fat Flush Plan, you may not experience any symptoms at all. But if you do feel tired, grouchy or headachy, don't lose heart. Realise that these symptoms are an indication that both the fast and the detox process are working and that you'll soon feel even better than you did before.

SKIP THE SUPPLEMENTS

No one is a bigger fan of vitamin, mineral and nutritional supplements than I am. But one time you should not take these otherwise highly recommended products is during a fast. Your body will have a hard time digesting even the finest dietary supplements on an empty stomach, and they might even make you nauseous. You can start taking your supplements again during the Three-Day Sequel, but please skip them during your One-Day Fast.

Onwards and Upwards

One of the most powerful aspects of fasting, I've found, is the way it helps you rethink your life and clarify your priorities. I was struck that Lucy, Nila and Jason all felt re-energised after their One-Day Fast, not only in regard to diet, but also as they thought about their lives.

Jason, for example, found himself thinking about how strong the fast had made him feel and when else he had felt that way. He made what I considered a powerful connection, discovering that whenever he was able to extend himself past what he thought were his limits and offer help to family, friends or colleagues, he experienced that same sense of strength. For him, the One-Day Fast was an opportunity to get in touch with an aspect of his personality that he had often tended to disregard.

Nila spent most of her fast day doing errands and tending to her children, as she had planned. When we first spoke, she described the day as uneventful, though she was relieved that she hadn't experienced either the hunger or the fatigue she had feared. Then she added, 'Because I wasn't giving myself food, I started to think about what else I needed during that busy day. Sometimes, I think my needs get lost in all the busy-ness. I don't know what I'll do about that, exactly, but I'm going to think about it.'

But it was Lucy who had the most exciting experience. She came bounding into my office, saying triumphantly, 'I did it! One whole day without food!' For Lucy, who had always experienced herself as a needy, dependent person, it was liberating to find out that she had more internal resources than she thought. 'Besides,' she said with a grin, 'when I did start eating again, the food tasted *sooooo* good!'

The Miracle Juice was very filling. Only when I had gaps in sipping did I notice a slight want for food. I noticed a slight increase in my energy level and, by the end of the day, the swelling in my ankles had disappeared!

– PATRICIA A. APRE, AGE FIFTY; LOST 2.25 KG/5 LB

* Warning: Once you have concluded your One-Day Fast, be sure to continue on and complete the Three-Day Sequel. Fasting without proper follow-up can leave you feeling constipated, bloated and sluggish, and it can also sabotage your weight loss. Now that you've achieved the hardest part of the programme, make sure you seal in your results with the Three-Day Sequel.

YOUR FAST TRACKER LOG:
THE ONE-DAY FAST

The morning of the fast

My weight _____

MY MEASUREMENTS:

Waist_____

Thighs _____

The evening of the fast

What strategies worked for me today?

_____

_____

What will I do differently if I ever fast again?

_____

_____

How do I feel about the One-Day Fast?

_____

_____

The morning after the fast

My weight _____

MY MEASUREMENTS:

Waist_____

Thighs _____

Making the Most of Your Day: Emotional Detox

*Your vision will become clear only when you
look into your heart. Who looks outside, dreams.
Who looks inside, awakens.*

– CARL JUNG

Linda and I had spent several minutes going over the protocol for the Fast Track. An experienced dieter, she wasn't worried about following the Seven-Day Prequel or the Three-Day Sequel. But she was concerned about making it through her One-Day Fast.

'I'm really afraid of how hungry I'll get,' she kept saying.

I tried to reassure her, explaining that the Miracle Juice I had created was especially designed to forestall hunger pangs, balance blood sugar and offer a satisfying, lively taste. I told her about the experiences of other Fast

Trackers who had not only avoided feeling hungry but had also enjoyed unexpected surges of energy or benefited from a calm, alert feeling – a steady mental clarity that was the very opposite of the distraction and mental fog that comes from feeling hungry. I even shared my own experiences of one-day fasts. As the day wore on, I told her, I actually felt *less* interested in food, rather than more. I used the day as a kind of Sabbath, a day of rest to focus on my feelings, thoughts and priorities, a time to get clear about what I was really hungry for.

Linda listened politely, but I could see that nothing I said seemed to make much difference. Finally, on impulse, I said, 'Linda! What are you really worried about?'

Linda looked at me in distress. 'If I'm not eating, what will I *do* with myself all day?' she burst out.

It turned out that Linda, a busy fashion executive, used her weekend mealtimes as a major way to relax and socialise. Although she worked long, gruelling hours during the week and spent Saturday on a frantic round of errands (on the rare weekends when she didn't also have to log in some work time), Sunday was a time to power down and hang out with friends. A typical Sunday might start with a leisurely three-hour brunch, followed by drinks with her best friend and then a romantic dinner with her boyfriend. Although Linda didn't necessarily eat very much at any of these meals, she saw them as her only chance to just be. Even when she ate alone, she'd use the time to read, think and daydream, dawdling for hours in a pavement café or at her kitchen table at home.

'Terrific,' I said when I heard her explanation. 'Then this fast day will have an extra purpose for you. You'll get to find out all the other ways you can "just be" – ways that have nothing to do with food.'

After Linda left, I thought about all the ways the food in our lives is so much more than 'just food'. I, too, am what my highly respected colleague, counsellor and corporate consultant, Linda Spangle, calls an 'emotional eater', an eloquent phrase that she explains in her breakthrough book *Life Is Hard, Food Is Easy*. I've often used food as comfort, to help me relax, calm me down or ground me. Some of my warmest memories of family and friends are centred on the holiday meals we've shared or the hours we've spent just hanging out in the kitchen, nurtured by its cosiness during those long hard winters when I was living in Bozeman, Montana. And when I want to reach out to a friend in need – someone who's lost a loved one or suffered another tragedy – I turn to the age-old custom of bringing food.

There's nothing wrong with these responses; in fact, I think they're part of what makes us human. But one of the things I love about one-day fasts is the way they help us widen our horizons. Taking a break from eating – while nourishing our bodies with Miracle Juice and drinking lots of pure water – gives us new opportunities to indulge ourselves in other ways. Once we're not using food for comfort, pleasure and relaxation, we have the chance to find out what other ways we can have fun, pamper ourselves or enjoy a much-needed break.

Mindful that fasting can be an exciting and perhaps

somewhat scary experience for those who have not tried it before, I'm using this chapter to provide you with some emotional and practical support for your fasting day. However you choose to spend it, I know it will be one of your happiest and most satisfying days in a long time. Here are a few suggestions that may make it even better. Browse through them and choose any or all that you think will work for you. Or craft your own special fast day. I wish you luck on your journey!

Conscious Breathing

Conscious breathing is a technique that enables you to become more aware and present with every breath. It's a wonderful way to ground yourself, to relax, to get in touch with your true feelings or to make a little oasis of calm in the midst of a frantic day. Conscious breathing can be done for as little as two minutes or as much as thirty minutes at a time – while you're stuck in a traffic jam, as part of a lunch hour or instead of a short nap. On trips to New York, I've even done a bit of conscious breathing in the subway! It's a wonderful way to both calm down and restore your system with energising oxygen – a nutrient that we are often deprived of in our busy, stressful, shallow-breathing world. If you're concerned about overeating, conscious breathing is a terrific way to begin a meal; take a two- to five-minute 'focus time' to connect you to your body and release the stress that can interfere with the production of stomach acid, making you more conscious of every bite you take and of how full you are becoming. On today, your fast day, you can indulge in conscious breathing for five minutes at a time to combat hunger pains, or engage in longer sessions as a consciousness-raising experience. Once you master this simple technique, you may start to wonder how you ever got along without it.

COPING WITH HUNGER

The many Fast Trackers who have tried the One-Day Fast reported remarkably few hunger pangs during their time without food. But every so often, you might feel a twinge, whether it's physical hunger or simply the emotional sense that it's time for you to eat. Here are some suggestions to help you make it through those times:

- *Sip some Miracle Juice or water.* The juices and spices in the Miracle Juice will help ease any physical symptoms of hunger you experience, including low blood sugar. Both the juice and the water will help you feel full.

- *Focus on the feeling.* Often our experience of hunger is an emotional one, linked to powerful feelings of grief, sadness, anger, joy, pleasure and love. Use one of the conscious-breathing exercises or suggestions for journal writing given in this chapter to uncover your associations with food and get in touch with your 'true' hunger.

* *Give yourself a (non-food) treat.* Often we become so used to rewarding ourselves, relaxing or re-energising with food that we lose track of other means to fill these important needs. Because you're not eating today, you've got lots of time to do other things – so what else might you enjoy? Here are some possibilities – can you think of others?

a relaxing walk

writing in your journal

watching a video

talking to a friend

reading an absorbing book

getting a manicure, pedicure or facial

going for a massage (be sure to ask the masseur to use only natural oils)

soaking in the bath, with scented oils and candles

painting, drawing, moulding clay

listening to music

dancing (by yourself is okay)

doing a craft project, such as knitting or crocheting

* *Try some conscious breathing.* Deep breathing feeds our bodies with oxygen. If we got more of the 'breath of life', I have the feeling none of us would be so hungry. Conscious breathing also expands our awareness of our bodies, and helps

us connect to feelings of joy and calm. (I've offered some suggestions for conscious breathing in this chapter.)

Conscious Breathing: The Preparation

1. Start by choosing a quiet, peaceful place where you can conduct this exercise. Turn off the radio and the TV and unplug the phone. Just as you are allowing your stomach to be free of food, you will allow your environment to be free of noise – or at least, of noise that makes particular demands on you.

2. Set aside at least five minutes to start. I recommend setting a timer, so that you can focus entirely on your breathing without looking at the clock.

3. Sit in a comfortable position with your feet flat on the floor. Don't lie down – you might fall asleep! Your back should be straight and well supported. The goal is to be alert and present, but relaxed. Let your hands rest loosely in your lap or on your knees. Don't fold your hands or cross your feet; this exercise works better when each part of your body remains relatively separate.

4. Close your eyes and begin to breathe. Ideally, you should be breathing in on a slow count of eight and breathing out on the same count. If you find it difficult to breathe that slowly, don't worry. Breathe in a slow count of two, and out on two. When you are comfortable with that speed,

breathe in on four and out on four. Continue adding time to each inhale and exhale as you feel comfortable, until you've worked your way up to an inhale of eight counts and an exhale of eight counts. If the idea of slowing your breath even further attracts you, go ahead, but eight is slow enough for the exercise to work.

5. Allow your abdomen to expand as your breath fills your diaphragm. Many of us are used to 'chest breathing', so that our lungs expand and contract with every breath. That's terrific, but for this exercise you also want to 'belly breathe'. If you're not sure what this means, place one hand gently on your abdomen. Feel your abdomen expand, like a balloon filling up, as you breathe in. Feel it collapse, like a balloon letting out air, as you breathe out. If you're not used to breathing this way, it may take you a while – even the entire five minutes – to get comfortable with it. Or you may feel comfortable right away. Either way, just take your time and breathe. Don't force your breath. Think of the breath as floating in and floating out. Rather than pushing or pulling, you are simply allowing the breath to enter and leave your body.

Once you're comfortable with the slow, regular belly breathing I've just described, you can begin to allow your consciousness to open as well. You have several choices. You can simply continue to breathe, slowly and calmly, focusing entirely on the process of breathing. Or you can engage in any one of the following journeys. Make a tape of your voice talking you through this process or simply let your own mind guide you.

Conscious Breathing: The Journey

OPTION 1: MY BREATH, MY BODY, MYSELF

I breathe in and feel my breath filling my lungs. I follow my breath as it travels down into my diaphragm. I'm with my breath as it filters into my blood and flows throughout my body. As my breath expands, it fills me all the way up to my skin. When I breathe out, I release everything I do not need. I feel my breath travel inwards from my skin, through my blood, back into my diaphragm, up through my lungs. I let it go. Then there is room for a new breath, filling my lungs. I follow my breath as it travels down into my diaphragm . . .

(Continue with this exercise, allowing your awareness of your body to expand with every breath.)

OPTION 2: WHOLE-BODY BREATHING

As I breathe in, I feel the breath begin at the soles of my feet, where they are grounded against the floor. The breath travels up my legs, my thighs, my abdomen, my chest, my shoulders, my throat, my head and up to the crown of my skull, where I feel it connect to the universe beyond me. Then I release the breath, feeling all tension release with it, down through my face, my neck, my spine, my hips, my thighs, my calves, my ankles and out through my feet into the ground. When I breathe in again, the breath begins again at the soles of my feet . . .

(Continue with this exercise, allowing your awareness of your body to become more specific with every breath. This is a terrific way to identify and then release tension.)

OPTION 3: BREATHE IN THE GOOD, RELEASE THE BAD

As I breathe in, I draw in [choose an element you would like to connect to; it could be energy, light, love, joy, peace, contentment or any other positive force or emotion]. I feel [this good thing] moving through my body with the breath. I feel it filling my lungs, my heart, my stomach. I enjoy and savour [this good thing]. As I breathe out, I release [whatever emotion or experience you would like to release, such as fear, worry, anger, confusion, stress or hunger]. I feel the breath drawing all [the emotion/experience] from my body, from my arms, my legs, my stomach, my head, my chest, my heart. As I breathe out, I release [the emotion/experience] completely. [Continue to repeat this exercise with every breath. This can be an emotional exercise, and I advise you to simply let the emotions flow. If you feel tearful or find yourself beginning to cry, continue to breathe as slowly and evenly as possibly, letting the grief flow through you. If you find yourself feeling sudden anger or frustration, experience the feeling while continuing to breathe. I've often noticed that doing this exercise moves me through 'negative' emotions to a place of joy and peace, but the key is to allow the emotions to keep flowing. The discipline of a slow, steady breath keeps you safe and grounded while your emotions are released. And if you do find yourself crying, make sure to drink a nice, big glass of water afterwards. Nothing is more sooth-ing for your body and spirit.]

My complexion is better, and I had a wonderful sleep last night. I learned more about myself, and how I can eat to feel better about myself. I would definitely do this again because it's a terrific detox and my body feels so good today. And this is just the first day!

– CRYSTAL FRASER, TWENTY-SIX; LOST 2.5 KG/5½ LB

Sealing in the Results: The Three-Day Sequel

The reward for work well done is the opportunity to do more.

– JONAS SALK

* Warning: You *must* follow the One-Day Fast with this Three-Day Sequel, or your re-entry into normal eating might leave you more bloated, constipated and 'toxic' than you were before. Fasting without follow-up support means that the toxins released into your bloodstream during the fast may remain in your system, making you feel tired, anxious, headachy and more fatigued than when you started. You'll also be likely to gain more weight.

Sealing in the Results of Your Fast

Miriam was a short, intense woman in her early fifties who had struggled with weight loss since she'd gone into early menopause in her mid-forties. When she heard about the Fast Track, she was thrilled, particularly after I suggested that its special Seven-Day Prequel, Miracle Juice and Three-Day Sequel might actually rev up her metabolism and make it easier for her to keep the weight off.

THE FAST TRACK SEQUEL – THREE DAYS

Seal in the results of your one-day fast with the eight simple steps that are described here.

I. EACH DAY, CHOOSE AT LEAST ONE OF THE FOLLOWING PROBIOTIC FOOD SOURCES TO RESTORE 'FRIENDLY BACTERIA':

- sauerkraut (90 g/3 oz): you can either make your own sauerkraut or buy an organic, raw variety. Most shop-bought sauerkraut is processed with heat, which kills the naturally occurring enzymes and microflora; so check the label very carefully.
- yoghurt (240 ml/8 fl oz): non-fat, low-fat or whole-milk yoghurt are all fine, but look for natural yoghurt whose label reads 'active and live active cultures'.

II. BEFORE EACH MEAL, TAKE 1 OR MORE TABLETS OF HYDROCHLORIC ACID IN A FORMULA THAT CONTAINS AT LEAST 300 TO 325 MILLIGRAMS OF BETAINE HYDROCHLORIDE WITH AT LEAST 130 MILLIGRAMS OF PEPSIN, AND 50 MILLIGRAMS OF OX BILE EXTRACT.

III. EACH DAY, CHOOSE AT LEAST ONE LIVER-LOVING FOOD FROM EACH GROUP:

1. **The Crucifers** (40 g/1½ oz)
   cabbage, cauliflower, broccoli

2. **Green Leafy Vegetables and Herbs** (60 g/2 oz)
   parsley, kale, watercress, chard, coriander, beet-root tops, endive

3. **Citrus** (1 orange or juice of ½ a lemon or lime)
   orange, lemon, lime

4. **Sulphur-Rich Foods**
   garlic (at least one clove, finely chopped), onions (60 g/2 oz), eggs (2)

5. **Liver Healers**
   artichoke (1 small artichoke or 4 cooked artichoke hearts), asparagus (5 medium spears, cooked), beetroot (145 g/5 oz), dandelion root tea (1 to 2 cups)

IV. Each day, choose at least two of the following Colon-Caring Foods: milled or ground flaxseeds (2 to 3 tablespoons), carrot (I small raw), apple (I small raw with skin), pear (I small raw with skin)

V. Each day, drink half your body weight in ounces of filtered or purified water.

VI. Each day, make sure you have at least two servings (the size of the palm of your hand) of protein in the form of lean beef, veal, lamb, skinless chicken, turkey or fish, or, if you're a vegan or vegetarian, at least 2 tablespoons a day of a high-quality blue-green algae or spirulina source.

VII. Each day, make sure you have I to 2 tablespoons of oil in the form of olive oil, flaxseed oil or Woman's Oil (a flaxseed oil-blackcurrant-seed oil blend).

VIII. Avoid the following Detox Detractors:
- excess fat, especially trans fats from margarine, and processed and fried foods

- sugar and all its relatives, including high-fructose corn syrup, honey, molasses, sugar cane crystals, pure sugar cane juice, evaporated cane juice, dried cane juice, maltodextrin and all products ending in '-ose' (such as sucrose, dextrose, fructose and levulose)
- artificial sweeteners, including aspartame, sucralose or Splenda, and sugar alcohols (such as maltitol, mannitol, sorbitol and xylitol)
- refined carbohydrates, including white rice and products made from white flour
- gluten, found in wheat, rye, barley and all their products (including bread, pasta, crackers), also found in many 'low-carb' products (such as packaged cereals, macaroni cheese, pizza-dough mix, spaghetti, shells, tortillas, pancake/waffle mixes and biscuits), and in vegetable proteins, modified food starch, some soy sauces and distilled vinegars
- soya protein isolates, found in low-carb 'energy' bars, and soya protein powders; and processed soya foods (such as soya milk, soya cheese, soya ice cream, soya hot dogs and soya burgers)
- alcohol; over-the-counter drugs; and caffeine, including coffee, tea, fizzy drinks and chocolate
- mould, found on overly ripe fruits, especially melons, bananas and tropical fruits.

Miriam had no problem following the Seven-Day Prequel – an intelligent and well-read person, she well understood the need for supporting the liver and colon before beginning a fast. And when she lost 2.25 kg/5 lb on her One-Day Fast, she was delighted.

Then came the Three-Day Sequel. Happy with the results she'd already enjoyed, Miriam decided to skip the follow-up to the fast. When I saw her a week later, she had gained back half the weight she'd lost, and she was suffering from constipation and bloating. I asked her about how closely she'd followed the Fast Track protocol. Blushing, she admitted that she'd failed to complete the Three-Day Sequel.

'I felt like I was done,' she told me. 'I didn't really see the need to keep going.'

Because she was already so frustrated and uncomfortable, I didn't have the heart to scold her. I gave her some suggestions for adding fibre to her diet, and sent her on her way. But her experience reminded me just how important it is to give yourself the proper nutritional support *after* your fast as well as before. Undergoing the Fast Track is a wonderful opportunity to unclog your colon and begin detoxing your system. But if you don't follow up with extra colon and liver support – and particularly with extra fibre to bind the toxins you have released through your weight loss – you could end up in worse shape than before you began.

So let's take a closer look at the Three-Day Sequel. As I hope you've realised by now, every single step of this programme is there for a reason – to support your weight loss and your health. If you skip any aspect of the programme, you'll only be cheating yourself.

Ease Back into Eating

My first suggestion is that you ease back into eating by choosing cooked, low-fat foods that are easy to digest. For breakfast, for example, try the Morning-After Puffy Apple Flaxcake, for which you'll find a recipe in Chapter 8. This recipe contains both high-fibre flaxseed and pectin-rich apple, which both bind up toxic wastes and help elimination. If possible, have this pancake for breakfast your first day – or even all three days of the Sequel to get things moving. (You will note that the Morning-After Puffy Apple Flaxcake already contains two sources of fibre so you may not need to choose an additional fibre source that day. Or you might – you will know how you feel.)

TAKE IT SLOW AND EASY

Keep in mind that how you break the fast is just as important as the fast itself. And the way you eat is just as important as what you eat. So, first and foremost, because digestion begins in the mouth, you must eat slowly and chew your food very well. Try to chew about thirty times per bite.

Of course, you shouldn't overeat – less is more when you're breaking a fast. And make your transition into your post-fast eating by sticking with light and easy-to-digest foods, as well as focusing on cooked foods rather than raw (it's easier on the digestion).

Finally, keep the food combinations simple. Use this time as an opportunity to appreciate how good food tastes when you haven't eaten for an entire day and how nourishing your new food choices will be for your 3 trillion cells.

Keep your choices very basic, especially for the first day. Go for foods in simple combinations. Don't eat fruit and vegetables in the same meal because these foods require different sets of enzymes to digest and, after a fast, that can cause *in*digestion in sensitive systems. You should also choose just one protein per meal. This could be accompanied by a soup or some steamed or puréed veggies. Save your fruit to eat by itself, as a snack.

I've suggested this transition period as a safeguard to your health. But you might also want to use this time to savour the smells, tastes and textures of the food you eat. Choose foods with bright, rich colours, such as steamed red peppers, yellow squash and purple cabbage. Besides being pleasing to the eye, the intense colour also indicates the presence of *flavonoids*, powerful anti-oxidants that will both nourish your liver and fight the ageing process. Keep your portions small, especially for the first day. This is an opportunity to discover how much – or how little – you need to feel full, particularly when you are savouring every bite.

Making Friends with Bacteria

You've already noticed that I started this Three-Day Sequel by instructing you to consume probiotics in the form of sauerkraut or yoghurt, fermented foods that will help restore friendly bacteria to your system. The use of these probiotic fermented foods is perhaps one of the most important, and most overlooked, aspects of nutrition, and one that will be a particular problem for any of you who've been on a low-carb, high-protein diet. Whenever you eat heavy-duty amounts of protein and cheese from non-organically raised animals, you are unknowingly ingesting second-hand antibiotics that are contained in all that conventionally farmed beef, chicken or pork – antibiotics that are equal-opportunity drugs and kill off all your bacteria, too, even the friendly ones on which your body depends.

As we saw earlier, our intestinal tracts are full of 'friendly bacteria' whose job is to help us digest our food and to combat the unfriendly bacteria that cause disease. In our large bowel alone, some 100 trillion bacteria make their home, including more than 400 different species. They actually weigh about 1.4 kg/3 lb, but that's one type of weight you don't want to lose. Without these friendly flora, you couldn't synthesise vitamins, break down toxins or digest fibre – they're the ones who break down indigestible plant materials into the short-chain fatty acids on which your colon cells desperately rely. They also help transport nutrients, produce lactase and other enzymes to help you digest milk sugars and help in the synthesis of vitamin K and all the B vitamins.

Your liver is also happy when friendly bacteria are flourishing, because some research indicates that a shortage of beneficial bacteria is correlated with cirrhosis and diabetes. And new studies suggest that friendly bacteria may offer a host of other benefits, including helping you digest fats, proteins and carbohydrates, and controlling excess LDL or 'bad' cholesterol levels.

The weight-loss advantage of such elements is clear. But perhaps most useful of all for your weight loss is understanding that when your body is finally digesting and absorbing nutrients at peak efficiency, you won't be nearly so hungry. You'll be able to eat far less food, with far greater satisfaction.

WHO ARE THE GOOD BACTERIA?

If you're welcoming the friendly bacteria into your system, you should probably know them by name! The two main categories are called *lactobacillus* and *bifido* bacterium. The lactobacilli hang out in your small intestines, while the bifido bacteria live in the large intestines. These tiny organisms prevent damage to the lining of your gastrointestinal tract and help crowd out the really bad or pathogenic bacteria (like the infamous *Escherichia coli*) by creating a 'barrier wall' in your intestines. By keeping in check disease causing microbes, probiotics are your immune system's best friends. These good bacteria may also be the newest weapon in the fight against cancer, balancing glucose and lipid levels and helping ward off osteoporosis.

Good vs. Bad Bacteria: A Balance of Power

Your small intestine is the home of 60 per cent of your immune system, which literally resides in the lining of this key organ. When you consider that for most of human history, the biggest dangers to our health would have come from eating poisonous food, it makes sense that our bodies are designed for a quick first-line response whenever something unhealthy enters our intestinal tract. This immune response largely depends on good bacteria – another reason why it's so important to promote their growth.

The problem, of course, comes from the fact that many of the same conditions friendly to good bacteria also provide a breeding ground for bad bacteria and other life forms, including parasites and yeast. And, by the same token, the antibiotics (literally, 'anti-life' medications) that destroy bad bacteria and the treatments that rid you of yeast infections are also likely to kill off good bacteria.

In the healthy intestinal system, good bacteria, bad bacteria and yeast create a kind of balance of power, in which all three life forms live within you, with the good bacteria free to do its healthy work. Ideally, you want a ratio of 85 per cent friendly bacteria to 15 per cent unfriendly bacteria. Killing off the good bacteria upsets the balance of power in your internal ecology, however, leaving room for the yeast to get out of control, with such symptoms as bloating, gas, diarrhoea, eczema, hives and even psoriasis.

If you've been taking antibiotics, you need to make sure that you're also taking *probiotics* at the same time and for at least two months thereafter to restore the balance of bacterial power. By the same token, now that you've completed two-thirds of the Fast Track, you need to replenish your friendly bacteria. By detoxifying your system – particularly if you were successful at freeing your colon from any faecal encrustation that built up along its walls – you've also made life far more difficult for the friendly bacteria within your gut. So in this Three-Day Sequel, we're going to start building up those helpful bacteria. This is where both sauerkraut (fermented cabbage) and yoghurt (fermented milk) come into the health picture.

Sauerkraut is a natural source of lactic acid, a highly beneficial organic acid that results from the fermentation or culturing of foods. Of all the organic acids formed during the fermentation process, lactic acid is the most powerful inhibitor of the type of bacteria that causes putrefaction in the gut; yet it never makes your system overly acid.

Sauerkraut is such a healing food that, during the American Civil War, when the 'soured cabbage' was added to prisoners' diets, smallpox death rates plummeted from 90 per cent to only 5 per cent. Although you probably don't have to worry about smallpox today, you can imagine the beneficial effect of this common food on the nasty bacteria in your own system. Sauerkraut is a rich source of *Lactobacillus plantarum*, a potent strain of friendly bacteria that gives *Candida*, *Salmonella*, *E. coli* and parasites the heave-ho.

You can make your own vitamin-, fibre- and enzyme-rich sauerkraut (see Ann Louise's Home-Made Sauerkraut, at the end of this book) or buy it ready-made in your local health-food shop. But again make sure that the sauerkraut you buy is raw, because cooking sauerkraut kills the enzymes and microflora that you need to restore the friendly bacteria.

THE FAST TRACK PROBIOTIC WAY

If you are still not a sauerkraut fan, even after you've tried my fabulous Home-Made Sauerkraut, and if yoghurt isn't your idea of high-culture cuisine, there are supplement options which you can find in the complete *Fast Track Detox Diet*. (Century.)

Yoghurt is also a tried and true food source of probiotics, chock full of lactobacilli, but only if it's made with live active cultures. It's been used for centuries to help digestive problems, stop diarrhoea, enhance immunity and fight off infection because of its high content of the lactobacilli and *L. thermophilus* strain of friendly bacteria. Cow, goat and sheep yoghurt are all available and each is a healthy choice, but steer clear of frozen yoghurt – freezing kills the live cultures. Make sure whatever yoghurt you buy says 'made with active and live cultures' on the label.

Helpful Hydrochloride

Now that you've cleansed so many toxic wastes from your system, you need to make sure that no more toxins accumulate from putrefying proteins or undigested food. A little HC1 taken before meals will help your stomach acids do their job – a particularly necessary supplement if you've been on a low-carb diet, which tends to overload your system with proteins that deplete your stomach acids. One of the nice things about adding HC1 is that it's one of the very few inorganic acids that is a normal constituent of the body anyway, so you can't lose by adding a bit more. And if there's extra ox bile in your HC1 supplement, as I recommend, you'll get a boost in digesting fat and promoting peristalsis, that undulating motion in the small intestine that leads to proper elimination. Remember, I recommend a supplement that includes 300 to 325 milligrams of betaine hydrochloride, 130 milligrams of pepsin and 50 milligrams of ox bile.

Fun with Fibre

As we've seen, keeping your fibre content high is super-important in this Three-Day Sequel. You need fibre to bind up the toxins you've released and to keep food moving through your system. I strongly recommend the Morning-After Puffy Apple Flaxcake for your first breakfast as a food source that includes both soluble and insoluble fibre – and is light and filling, to boot. You may enjoy it so much that you have it all three days! And because this breakfast dish is so fibre-rich, you don't need to choose any other fibre source for that day.

It's especially important to chew fibrous foods slowly and carefully. If you're getting your fibre in the form of apples, carrots, celery or berries, make sure you chew each bite thoroughly. You can try counting to twenty-five on every chew before you swallow. Or simply focus on the amazing tastes that are released into your mouth with every bite. For these post-fast meals, try not to do anything while you eat except focus on the food, no reading, watching TV or even talking. Concentrate on the delicious sensations that even the humblest meal can offer you, and marvel at Nature's bounty of fruit, vegetables, herbs and spices.

Don't Forget the Water!

By now you've been drinking so much water, you may feel as though you're ready to float away! But don't stop drinking. You really need the excess fluids to keep the toxins flowing *out* of your body, as well as to keep food moving through your bowels. The worst possible time to cut back on water is in the three days after a fast – that's when your system needs more lubrication than ever, particularly because you are also keeping up your fibre intake, which can have a dehydrating effect.

Looking Towards the Next Level

Now that you've completed your time on the Fast Track, I hope you've both lost some weight and gained a new attitude. I'll make a small confession here: I didn't want you to try detox just for the eleven days it took to complete the Fast Track. My real agenda was for you to become so hooked on detox that you'd start to eat healthy, clean, organic foods; cleanse your system regularly; and discover that the best way to lose weight and to keep it off is to protect your health, your body and our planet.

What you'll do from here is up to you. But if you'd like some guidance on how to take the Fast Track to the next level, you will find everything you need to know in the complete *Fast Track Detox Diet* – whether you're looking for another quick fix after your next holiday splurge, or a lifelong devotion to clean, healthy and delicious food.

Usually I'm tired and don't get much done at home. But on my fast day, I took a long, slow walk, then cleaned the house and did five loads of washing. 'Wow,' I said to myself. 'It's 11.45 at

*night and I'm not tired yet.' At lunch, I wasn't hungry even
after my daughter ate a double cheeseburger and fries right in
front of me. Wow!!! I plan on using your One-Day Detox Diet
again – because it works! I love not feeling tired all day. I feel
rejuvenated and more focused. I love the abundance of energy –
and I love seeing my chin back.*

– BEVERLY GRZEJKA, FIFTY-SEVEN; LOST 1.9 KG/4¼ LB

YOUR FAST TRACKER LOG: THE SEQUEL

DAY ONE

I. The probiotics I ate today
1. _____
Others: _____

II. The Liver-Loving Foods I ate today
1. _____
2. _____
3. _____
4. _____
5. _____
Others: _____

III. The Colon-Caring Foods I ate today
1. _____
2. _____
Others: _____

IV. The water I drank today

I need to drink _____ ml/fl oz

Today I drank _____ ml/ fl oz of water

V. Today I did/did not avoid all detox detractors.

My evaluation

How do I feel about how I stuck to the Fast Track today?

_____

_____

What strategies worked for me?

_____

_____

What will I do differently tomorrow?

_____

_____

DAY TWO

I. The probiotics I ate today

1. _____

Others: _____

II. The Liver-Loving Foods I ate today

1. _____

2. _____

3. _____

4. _____

5. _____

Others: _____

III. The Colon-Caring Foods I ate today

1. _____
2. _____

Others: _____

What will I do differently tomorrow?

_____

_____

DAY THREE

I. The probiotics I ate today

1. _____

More: _____

II. The Liver-Loving Foods I ate today

1. _____
2. _____
3. _____
4. _____
5. _____

More: _____

III. The Colon-Caring Foods I ate today

1. _____
2. _____

Others: _____
More? _____

IV. The water I drank today
I need to drink_____ ml/fl oz
Today I drank_____ml/fl oz of water

V. Today I did/did not avoid all Detox Detractors.

My evaluation
How do I feel about how I stuck to the Fast Track today?
_____
_____

What strategies worked for me?
_____
_____

What will I do differently tomorrow?
_____
_____

Recipes

You will find a large number of surprisingly tasty and healthy detox recipes which make it easy to integrate the Fast Track into everyday eating. To make things super convenient for you, many of the recipes are identified as Prequel and/or Sequel and they include both liver-loving and colon-caring choices.

There is only room for a few in this condensed version of the book, so I've just included some of my favourites.

Liver-Loving Recipes

GARLICKY GREENS WITH GINGER AND LEMON

4 servings * Prequel- and Sequel-friendly

Greens are cleansing and full of liver-loving chlorophyll, especially those bitter greens. To take out the bitterness, always use a bit of salt when cooking. The salt sweetens the greens quite nicely, removing the bitter taste.

> 3 tablespoons low-sodium chicken stock or olive oil
> 1 large bunch (about 455 g/1 lb) greens (kale, chard, beetroot tops), cut crosswise with stems removed
> 2 garlic cloves, finely chopped
> ⅛ teaspoon of powdered ginger
> Pinch of salt
> 2 tablespoons fresh lemon juice

1. Heat the stock in a sauté pan over a medium heat.
2. Add the greens, garlic, ginger and salt, stirring until the greens wilt, about 1½ minutes.
3. Remove from the heat and drizzle on the lemon juice.

ABSOLUTELY ARTICHOKE SOUP

2 servings * Prequel- and Sequel-friendly

This is absolutely delicious, and your liver (not to mention your family) will agree!

> 1 tablespoon chicken stock or olive oil
> 1 small onion, finely chopped
> 4 garlic cloves, finely chopped
> 1 400 g/14 oz can artichokes, rinsed, drained and chopped
> 480 ml/16 fl oz stock
> ½ teaspoon dried parsley
> ½ teaspoon dried basil

½ teaspoon dried oregano
Salt to taste (optional)
Cayenne pepper to taste (optional)
Fresh lemon juice to taste (optional)

1. Heat the tablespoon of stock in a stockpot over a medium heat.
2. Sauté the onion and garlic until translucent.
3. Stir in the artichokes, stock and herbs. Add the salt, cayenne pepper and/or lemon juice, if using.
4. Cover and simmer for 30 minutes.

Colon-Caring Recipes

FLAXY CHICKEN WITH CITRUS RELISH

4 servings * Prequel- and Sequel-friendly

A little bit more involved in terms of time. But for those who love to cook, this recipe is loaded with fibre and is good for your waistline, too.

Citrus Relish

2 tablespoons grated orange zest
240 ml/8 fl oz fresh orange juice
1 teaspoon grated lime zest
2 tablespoons fresh lime juice
1 tablespoon arrowroot
1 orange, cut and sectioned like a grapefruit
100 g/3½ oz cucumber, seeded and diced
30 g/1 oz spring onions, chopped

30 g/1 oz yellow pepper, finely diced
30 g/1 oz red pepper, finely diced
2 tablespoons chopped coriander
Salt to taste
Cayenne pepper to taste

Chicken

Olive-oil spray
1 egg, beaten
4 tablespoons Dijon mustard
Salt (optional)
Cayenne pepper to taste
8 tablespoons milled or ground flaxseeds
4 boneless chicken breast halves, skin removed
1½ tablespoons olive oil

Citrus Relish

1. Combine the orange zest, orange juice, lime zest, lime juice and arrowroot in a small saucepan.
2. Simmer over a medium heat until bubbly and thick.
3. Cool.
4. In small bowl, mix the remaining relish ingredients. Stir in the orange and lime mixture until well blended.
5. Let the mixture stand, covered, for at least 1 hour so the flavours can marry.

Chicken

1. Preheat the oven to 180°C/350°F, Gas 4. Lightly coat a baking sheet with olive-oil spray.
2. Place the beaten egg in shallow dish.

3. Combine the mustard, salt (if using), cayenne pepper and flaxseeds in a pie dish.
4. Dip the chicken breasts into the beaten egg, and then dredge in the flaxseeds, coating all sides well.
5. Place the chicken on the baking sheet; drizzle with the olive oil.
6. Bake for 35 minutes, until the chicken is cooked through and the juices run clear.
7. Serve the chicken topped with the citrus relish.

PERFECT MUESLI

I serving * Prequel- and Sequel-friendly

This dish is my Fast Track version of the famous Bircher-Benner Muesli from Switzerland. This is suitable for people who want their fibre but do not need to lose weight.

2 tablespoons old-fashioned rolled oats (not instant)
juice of ½ lemon
I tablespoon whey in I tablespoon of filtered water
I medium pear
I tablespoon unprocessed, raw honey
2 tablespoons milled or ground flaxseeds, or chopped nuts of your choice

1. Soak the oats overnight in 4 tablespoons of filtered water.
2. In the morning, add the lemon juice and the whey mixture, blending well.
3. Grate the pear into the mixture.

4. Add the honey and flaxseeds and stir. Eat at once.

MORNING-AFTER PUFFY APPLE FLAXCAKE

1 serving * Prequel- and Sequel-friendly

This is definitely the breakfast of choice for the morning after the One-Day Fast. You can use this, of course, anytime in the programme.

1 egg
4 tablespoons grated apple
3 tablespoons milled or ground flaxseeds
⅛ to ½ teaspoon cinnamon
Olive oil spray

1. Whisk the egg, apple and flaxseed together with 1 to 2 tablespoons of filtered water in a small bowl.
2. Lightly coat an omelette pan with olive-oil spray and heat over a medium heat.
3. Pour the egg mixture into the pan and cook until the bottom of the flaxcake is solid enough to flip, 3 to 4 minutes.
4. Carefully flip the flaxcake, cooking until done, about 1 minute.
5. Sprinkle with the cinnamon and serve.

Probiotic-Powering Recipes

Featuring Sauerkraut and Yoghurt

ANN LOUISE'S HOME-MADE SAUERKRAUT

Makes 340 g/12 oz * Sequel-friendly

The key to this sauerkraut recipe is that it maintains its naturally occurring enzymes and microfloria. This is an uncooked rendition that is quite tasty.

150 g/5½ oz shredded red cabbage
150 g/5½ oz shredded green cabbage
1 teaspoon dried mustard
1 teaspoon caraway seeds
1 teaspoon salt
1 garlic clove, finely chopped
2 tablespoons fresh lemon juice

1. In a glass container with a lid, combine the cabbage, mustard, caraway seeds and salt.
2. In a separate small bowl, combine the garlic, lemon juice and 240 ml/8 fl oz filtered water. Then pour the mixture over the cabbage.
3. Cover tightly. Set aside and keep at room temperature for at least 3 days, shaking occasionally.

Blended Salad Recipes

It is very important the veggies in these blended salads are from organic vegetables. The last thing you want in your system is liquefied pesticides, sprays and fungicides.

GODDESS GREENS

1 serving

115 g/4 oz mixed green lettuce
2 celery sticks
30 g/1 oz spinach
1 cucumber
½ garlic clove, finely chopped (optional)
Juice of ½ lemon or lime

1. Cut the lettuce, celery, spinach and cucumber into small pieces.
2. Place the veggies and garlic, if using, in a food processor or blender. Process or blend until liquefied.
3. Add the lemon juice.
4. Drink immediately.

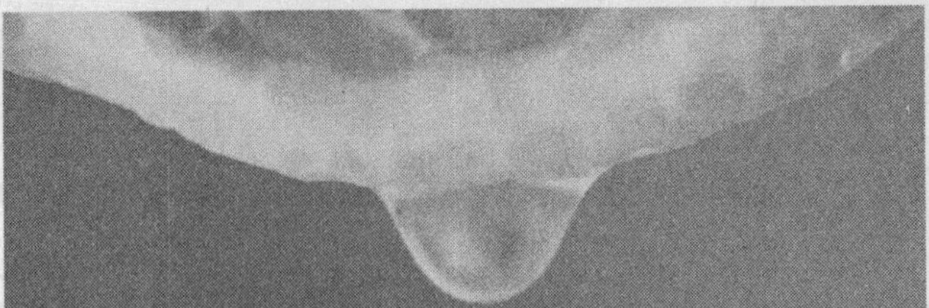

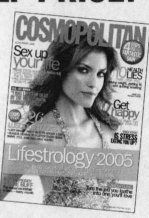